PARTNERSHIPS BETWEEN HEALTH
AND LOCAL GOVERNMENT

BOOKS OF RELATED INTEREST

REGULATING LOCAL AUTHORITIES
Emerging Patterns of Central Control
Edited by Paul Carmichael and Arthur Midwinter

RENEWING LOCAL DEMOCRACY
The Modernisation Agenda in British Local Government
Edited by Lawrence Pratchett

LOCAL GOVERNMENT REORGANISATION
The Review and its Aftermath
Edited by Steve Leach

QUANGOS AND LOCAL GOVERNMENT
A Changing World
Edited by Howard Davis

FINANCING EUROPEAN LOCAL GOVERNMENTS
Edited by John Gibson and Richard Batley

THE POLITICAL EXECUTIVE
Politicians and Management in European Local Government
Edited by Richard Batley and Adrian Campbell

PARTNERSHIPS BETWEEN HEALTH AND LOCAL GOVERNMENT

Editors

STEPHANIE SNAPE
PAT TAYLOR

In Memory of Lyn Harrison

Routledge
Taylor & Francis Group

LONDON AND NEW YORK

First published in 2004 in Great Britain by
FRANK CASS AND COMPANY LIMITED
and in the United States of America by
FRANK CASS PUBLISHERS
Copyright © 2004 Frank Cass & Co. Ltd

This edition published 2012 by Routledge
2 Park Square, Milton Park, Abingdon, Oxfordshire OX14 4RN
711 Third Avenue, New York, NY 10017
Routledge is an imprint of the Taylor & Francis Group, an informa business

British Library Cataloguing in Publication Data

Partnership between health and local government
   1. Public health administration – Great Britain
   2. Local government – Great Britain 3. Medical
   policy – Great Britain 4. Great Britain – Social policy
   I. Snape, Stephanie II. Taylor, Pat
   353.6'0941

   ISBN 978-0-714-68425-3 (pb)

Library of Congress Cataloging-in-Publication Data

Partnerships between health and local government / editors, Stephanie
Snape, Pat Taylor.
     p. cm.

Includes bibliographical references and index.
   ISBN 0-7146-5537-6 (Cloth) -- ISBN 0-7146-8425-2 (Paper)
   1. Fundholding (Medical economics)--Great Britain--Citizen
participation. 2. Medical policy--
Great Britain--Citizen participation. I. Snape, Stephanie.
II. Taylor, Pat, 1948 May 15- III.
Local government studies. IV. Title.
   RA410.55.G7P37 2003
   362.1'0941--dc22   2003017596

This group of studies first appeared in a Special Issue of
Local Government Studies (ISSN 0300-3930), Vol.29, No.3 (Autumn 2003)
[Partnerships between Health and Local Government].

Contents

Partnerships between Health and Local
   Government: An Introduction   STEPHANIE SNAPE
                            and PAT TAYLOR   1

Joint Planning across the Health/Social
   Services Boundary since 1946   PAUL BRIDGEN   17

Conceptual Issues in Inter-Agency
   Collaboration   WENDY RANADE
            and BOB HUDSON   32

Joint Working: The Health Service   CAROLINE GLENDINNING
   Agenda   and ANNA COLEMAN   51

Health and Local Government Partnerships:
   The Local Government Policy Context   STEPHANIE SNAPE   73

The Health Action Zone Initiative:
   Lessons from Plymouth   MICHAEL COLE   99

Overcoming the Desire for Misunderstanding
   through Dialogue   PAUL HOGGETT   118

Leading and Managing at the Boundary:
   Perspectives Created by Joined Up
   Working   MIKE BROUSSINE   128

Partnerships between Health and Local
   Authorities: Concluding Remarks   PAT TAYLOR   139

Abstracts   141

Notes on Contributors   145

Index   147

Partnerships between Health and Local Government: An Introduction

STEPHANIE SNAPE and PAT TAYLOR

The theme of this collection of essays is partnerships between health and local government. Interest in partnerships, and the range of joint working and collaborative activities undertaken within them, is not new. Nor is discussion of the merits (or otherwise) of collaboration between the two sectors; indeed, it is one of the 'hoary chestnuts' of social policy. However, New Labour's rise to power in 1997 has re-kindled an avid, acute interest in this 'old perennial'. The government's emphasis on partnerships and collaboration was projected as a key element of the 'Third Way', New Labour's self-proclaimed political philosophy. It was promoted as an antidote to the perceived damage done by the competitive ethos and market philosophy of the Conservative era. Partnership working was in particular viewed as the most appropriate means of addressing successfully those endemic social ills of society: low educational standards, social exclusion, poor health and poverty. No one agency could tackle such obdurate problems; these 'wicked issues' cross organisational boundaries and require collaborative solutions.

New Labour's enthusiasm for partnership approaches spawned many government reports, a range of area-based partnership initiatives, new powers and duties, incentives to collaborate and much exhortation to joint working. And in 1998, as the agenda of collaboration was being introduced, the Economic and Social Research Council (ESRC) commissioned a seminar series focused on the issue of 'improving partnerships between health and local government'. The aim of the seminar series, organised by the Universities of Birmingham, Northumbria and the West of England, was to 'provide a forum to exchange knowledge, experience and ideas about the relationship between health and local authorities, to discuss effective models of joint working, and to facilitate collaborative research and publications'. This seminar series provided the genesis of this special issue. All of the articles are based on – and are developments from – papers presented during the series, which ran during 1999 and 2000. It is not the only publication derived from the series. A number of practitioner-focused articles were published in a special issue of *Local Governance* (Ranade, 2001). This should be seen as an essential companion volume to this collection of essays, which comprises the more academic contributions to the series. The organisers would also like to take this opportunity to thank the ESRC for its support for the seminar programme.

This volume is dedicated to the memory of Lyn Harrison, who died in March 2001. Lyn worked for nearly 20 years at the University of Bristol in the School of Advanced Urban Studies (SAUS) and latterly in the School of Policy Studies. She spent much of that time researching, publishing and teaching in the area of joint working between health and local authorities and was an active contributor to the academic debate on joint working long before it was a key policy driver. Lyn was the rapporteur for the first ESRC seminar in Bristol in March 2000 and delivered a concise and critical analysis of the current partnership working agenda as a fitting conclusion to the debates at that seminar. Her long experience of partnership working would have been immensely valuable to the academic community at this time when there is such a focus on the need to evaluate and establish clear indicators for the value of partnerships. Her ability to 'see the wood from the trees' as well as her loyalty, friendship and irreverent sense of humour is sadly missed by her colleagues at Bristol and within the organisations around the country in which she carried out her research and consultancy.

This introductory article seeks to provide what every teacher (and apt pupil) understands as the two key features of any introduction: an explanation and description of the *context* within which collaboration has yet again become a favoured activity in the public sector; and a clear *structural map* of the succeeding essays which form this special issue, which also signposts the key *arguments and evidence* to be presented by the various authors. The context for the special issue has been examined through exploring the interesting relationship between New Labour's emphasis on partnership working and the debates about the nature of New Public Management (NPM). New Labour's love affair with the partnership mode of governing has been pivotal in instigating a fundamental debate about the nature of the public sector (and its reform programme – the Modernisation Agenda) in the United Kingdom.

PARTNERSHIPS AND THE SEARCH FOR A SUCCESSOR TO NEW PUBLIC MANAGEMENT

Prior to 1997, academics had spent some years debating and refining the concept of NPM; a phrase which had been coined to describe a paradigm shift in public policy away from the 'Old Public Administration' of bureaucracy, hierarchy and monolithic state provision to a 'New Public Management' of an increasingly fragmented public sector, imbued with a managerialist culture and relationships based on competition and marketised notions of the 'customer'. Hood's 1991 article in *Public Administration* has been rightly described by McLaughlin (2002) as the 'classic' and 'seminal' elucidation of NPM. He identifies seven doctrinal components:

- Hands-on professional management;
- Explicit standards and measures of performance;
- Greater emphasis on output controls;
- Shift to disaggregation of units in the public sector;
- Shift to greater competition in the public sector;
- Stress on private-sector styles of management practice;
- Stress on greater discipline and parsimony in resource use.

As a concept NPM appeared to provide a useful description of the radical changes to the UK public sector. These began in the mid-1970s and intensified during the Thatcher administrations. However, NPM was not simply a UK phenomenon. Hood and others argued that it was an international paradigm shift. Certainly, the parallels to the 'steering not rowing' *Reinventing Government* movement in the United States were obvious (Osborne and Gaebler, 1992). And a strong case could be made for identifying NPM-style reform programmes in a range of other countries, including New Zealand, Australia and Canada.

In a relatively short space of time, NPM became a favoured concept of academics, commentators and practitioners alike. It was an attractive conceptual framework for academic work. And it provided a useful basis for demands by policy-makers for further change (see for example, OECD, 1987). But its pre-eminence was to be questioned by the election of New Labour in 1997. Did New Labour's policies 'fit' into the confines of NPM? Could NPM be amended to incorporate the Blairite approach? Or was a successor to NPM required?

The relationship between New Labour and NPM has been complicated and confused by Labour's attempts to evolve its own – distinct – political philosophy. A pre-election dalliance with 'stakeholder politics' evolved after the election into the Third Way. This concept was promoted both by Labour politicians and by one of the party's resident academics, Anthony Giddens (Blair, 1998; Giddens, 1998). Giddens argues that the Third Way represents the centre-left response to the social democracy of the old left and the neo-liberalism of the new right; a modernising movement of the centre which seeks to promote a mixed economy of provision and a social investment state. And, as with NPM, its advocates proclaim the Third Way as an international change programme.

While New Labour and its proponents were busy espousing the Third Way, other commentators were determining their own approaches to assessing the 'distinctiveness' of New Labour. Newman (2001), for example, prefers the term 'modernising governance' to explain and explore the distinctiveness of New Labour policy. She argues that although there are 'points of continuity' between NPM and modernisation – and NPM remains the 'dominant' organisational regime – there were also distinctive themes in the areas of partnership working, citizen participation and involvement of public sector staff. The crucial issue here is the pivotal role that the emergence of partnerships has played in the challenge to the dominance of NPM.

Newman's work reflects a general trend among academics and policy-makers to abandon the language of NPM post-1997, and instead to embrace (or re-embrace) the concept and language of 'governance'. The debate surrounding 'governance' is some years old now and is complicated by the many different interpretations and uses of the term (corporate governance, minimal state and so on). However, some uses of the term have a particular resonance to the post-1997 partnership policy context. For example, Rhodes' concept of the dominance of networks in governance is particularly relevant: 'governance refers to self-organising, interorganisational networks characterized by interdependence, resource exchange, rules of the game and significant autonomy from the state' (1997: 15).

And recently a group of policy-makers and academics in the UK has been working to develop the concept of governance in relationship to Moore's work on 'public value' (1995). Benington (2003) has been influential in this emerging debate and he argues that three ideological conceptions of 'governance' can be identified: traditional public administration, NPM and networked governance. The key differences between networked governance and NPM include: a continuously changing *context* compared to one which is competitive; a perspective of *population* diversity versus an atomised view; *strategies* shaped by civil society rather than producer-centred strategy; *governance* through networks and partnerships versus governance through markets; and pivotal in this conceptualisation of these competing paradigms is the differing theoretical basis, with networked governance founded on an evolving concept of 'public value' and NPM underpinned by the theories of new institutional economics (including public choice).

Others have ridden to the defence of NPM (Osborne and McLaughlin, 2002; Ferlie and Fitzgerald, 2002). Osborne and McLaughlin argue that Hood's exposition of NPM 'is too narrow' and that the concept is 'not a static phenomenon but an evolving one' (2002: 10–11). They argue that the state has moved through four distinctive periods during its development – with the last two stages being the 'welfare state' and the 'plural state' respectively. NPM is part of the latter state:

However, this did not end with the market-based model of Thatcher. From 1997 onwards, the 'New Labour' government has taken the development of the plural state a stage further. This has been away from a narrow focus on the marketisation of public services and towards an emphasis on community governance ... the debate about NPM has been broadened from the earlier narrow concern with marketisation to one which focuses upon governance as the pre-eminent task of public management. (10)

Despite these arguments, there would seem to be two inter-related areas of new Labour policies challenging the continuity of NPM. The first is the Labour government's emphasis on partnership working and collaboration between the public, private and voluntary sectors. The second area is closely linked to partnerships: the change in focus from a marketised, individualised notion of the 'customer' to collectivist notions of the 'citizen', 'community' and 'civil society'. And the link is clear in many of New Labour's reforms; the concepts of the citizen and the community were to be key symbolic participants within their new partnership initiatives.[1]

This represents fundamental divergence from the policies of preceding Conservative administrations. Although they introduced a number of partnership initiatives (Private Finance Initiative, Training and Enterprise Councils, Urban Development Corporations, the Single Regeneration Budget), the main thrust of their approach to public sector reform was privatisation, markets, competition and contracts. And, their model of working with voluntary and community organisations was essentially the same as with private organisations – as contracted service providers rather than as distinctive representations of the public as stakeholders.

While New Labour has retained many of the organisational forms of the previous administration, such as contracting, in terms of partnership working their policy of promoting partnerships has taken many forms. They have mobilised a wide range of mechanisms and activities to achieve their collaborative vision (this could be interpreted positively, following Stoker, 2002, and Ham, 1999, as New Labour 'testing' a range of 'levers' to achieve their ends or more negatively, following Snape, 2000). Figure 1 details the range of *levers* utilised by the two Labour administrations, including exhortation and rhetoric, structural reorganisation, new powers and duties, new partnership initiatives and so on. The levers identified in Figure 1 are a mix of attempts to encourage *voluntary* collaboration and central *prescription* and mandate. And this mix is one of the many contradictions apparent in the Government's approach to encouraging partnership working.

It is precisely in this area of 'contradiction and paradox' that Newman has provided a distinctive voice (2001, 2002). She argues that New

FIGURE 1

LEVERS FOR PARTNERSHIP WORKING

Lever	Methods	Examples
Exhortation and rhetoric	Constant emphasis on partnership working in government speeches and government documents.	'There will be no return to the old centralised command and control systems, which stifled innovation and responsibility, and we reject the creation of pointless internal markets. Instead we favour partnerships at local level, with investment tied to targets and measured outcomes, with national standards, but freedom to manage and innovate' (Blair, 1998: 15).
Structural reorganisation	Creating new organisations or reshaping existing ones with a key theme of collaboration and partnership working.	Regional Development Agencies; Regional Assembles; Primary Care Trusts (PCTs); Care Trusts.
New Powers and duties	**Health Act (1999)** brought in 'duty of partnership'. For LAs to contribute to health improvement plans and PCTs to be part of LSPs. **Local Government Act (2000)** includes a power of well-being for local authorities. **Health Act Flexibilities** (DOH 2000) – pooled budgets, delegated responsibility for services. **Health and Social Care Act (2001)** – created powers for Secretary of State to require local partners to work together.	Local authorities have a power of promoting well being and PCTs must promote health (as opposed to curing illness). Currently the key focus for these new powers is the integration of the health–social care interface.
Provision of central funding	Targeted funding in which collaboration is a requirement.	Partnership grant given to Social Services Departments.
Integration of strategies and plans	Central government pressure on public and other agencies to work closer together to integrate strategies and plans.	Increasing pressure from the centre on regional bodies to 'join up' and co-ordinate the range of regional strategies.

FIGURE 1 (cont.)

Lever	Methods	Examples
New partnership programmes	Strategic partnerships. Sectoral partnerships. Neighbourhood/Area based partnerships. (This categorisation is taken from Sullivan and Skelcher, 2002: 24).	Encouragement from central government for health bodies ad local authorities to integrate their strategic planning processes through the medium of the Community Strategy. Local Strategic Partnerships (LSPs); Regeneration partnerships; Health and Education Action Zones Connexions; Community safety partnerships Sure Start; Healthy Living Centres; New Deal.
Deregulation	Changes made to statutory regulatory framework to allow more flexibility particularly in relation to financial provision.	Budget flexibilities; Pooled budgets.
Incorporation of partnership theme within performance management	Collaborative activity as a key performance indicator.	Best Value; Commission for Health Improvement (CHI) soon to be redesignated Commission for Health Care Audit and Inspection (CHAI) in April 2004.
Accountability	Public seen as key partners as service users, communities and citizens.	Patient Forums relating to all Health Trusts, Public involvement required in all national service frameworks (NSFs), Citizen panels.
	Local authority role in monitoring health service provision.	Power of health scrutiny provides councils with legitimate right to oversee health service developments, as a way of countering the democratic deficit within the NHS.

Labour's approach to reforming the public sector and public services is fraught with contradiction; in particular, the contradiction between encouraging partnership working while intensifying centrally derived performance management systems and continuing to embrace competition. Newman's argument is very much echoed in a number of the articles presented here (see in particular Glendinning and Coleman, and Snape). The exhortation and commitment to collaborative working is unquestioned; the reality is far more complex, as a number of the contributions to this volume demonstrate for the area of health–local government collaboration.

To summarise, this debate about the demise or adaptation of NPM is clearly likely to continue at least while Labour is in power. However, there are key aspects of the current policy climate that do not fit easily into NPM. NPM was premised on the concept of competition and contracts within the public sector. In Hood's seven doctrinal components of NPM no mention is given to collaboration, networks, joint working or partnerships. And, in truth, the work of Osborne and McLaughlin is less than convincing in arguing for New Labour's approach to be subsumed within NPM. The Labour administrations' focus on collaboration between the public, private and third sector is not easily accommodated within NPM. And so the search for a successor to NPM can largely be laid at the feet of the growing emphasis on partnership working, within which the exhortations to greater collaboration between health and local government play an important part.

THE CONTENT AND THEMES OF THE SPECIAL ISSUE

The above debate about the changing nature of government (or governance) in the United Kingdom provides the broad context to this collection of essays. However, the focus of this volume is one particular area of partnership working, namely partnerships, collaboration and joint working between health and local government. And there are good reasons to focus on this area since, as Glendinning and Coleman argue below, 'pressures on NHS and local government to engage in collaborative working have been particularly intense' (page 55).

The NHS has developed primarily as a service addressing the need to cure illness and disease. Two factors have been critical in shaping political concerns in relation to the NHS. The first is demographic change, with an ageing population placing growing demands on health and social care services. The second is the increasing capacity of the NHS to develop more complex and expensive methods to treat illness and disease, resulting in political concerns about the cost of providing this care, particularly within hospital settings. Policies over the past 20 years have required the NHS to reduce the overall numbers of hospital beds while at the same time reducing hospital waiting lists. The result has been intense pressure on health organisations to redefine the boundaries relating to when patients need care within a hospital setting and when they can be cared for at home with support from community based health and social services.

Further complications occur because social care is provided by local authority social services and community health services through health staff attached to GP practices. This has led to debates and struggles between local authority social services and health in relation to 'bed blocking' and continuing health care for older people and those with chronic health needs. However, the debate concerning bed blocking is just one example of the tensions between health and social care. In truth, this particular arena of collaborative working has long provided commentators with a rich area of study of the interrelationship between multiple factors affecting joint working between health and local authorities. Indeed, Wistow and Hardy (1991) developed a theoretical framework identifying five significant types of obstacle to interagency working in health and social care:

- *Structural* – lack of co-terminosity and fragmented responsibilities;
- *Procedural* – different operational systems and planning cycles;
- *Financial* – different funding streams and budget cycles;
- *Professional* – a range of differences around values and roles;
- *Status and legitimacy* – particularly between elected and appointed status.

Little wonder then that Former Secretary of State for Health Frank Dobson's description of the relationship between health and social care as the 'Berlin Wall' of social policy rang so true with academics and practitioners alike.

In analysing the nature of this 'Berlin Wall', there are a number of key questions which run as themes throughout the special issue. For any student or practitioner of partnerships these are unsurprising, comprising as they do many of the recurring debates in collaboration. These key questions are:

- What do we mean by 'partnerships'? How do we define them?
- What is the nature of the relationship between health and local government?
- What are the 'boundaries' of joint working between health and local government?
- What are the barriers to successful joint working?
- What opportunities have been thrown up by partnership working?
- What progress has been made in developing collaborative relationships?
- What effective models of joint working can be identified?

- What is the relationship between accountability and partnership working?
- What are the prospects for partnership working?
- Why partnerships?

All of the articles in the special issue touch upon some of these questions. However, before we turn to summarise each of these articles in turn it is important to address the first question listed above: the definition of partnerships.

Defining 'partnerships' has proved to be a difficult and contentious task. Certainly there is no one consensus definition. In reality there is a wide range of related terms: some tend towards describing the structures which facilitate partnership working and others more precisely describe the activities which together constitute 'working in partnership'. In practice all the following terms are often used interchangeably: joint working; network or networking; joined-up thinking; joined-up government; joint planning; inter-agency collaboration; inter-professional working; co-ordination; collaboration and collaborative advantage; joint venture; strategic alliance; co-ordinated service delivery; co-operation; coalition; policy co-ordination; seamless services and so on. All these terms have very positive connotations, in contrast to 'conflict' and 'competition'. For example, '"collaboration" is taken to imply a very positive form of working in association with others for some form of mutual benefit' (Huxham, 1996: 1).

In their recent analysis and mapping of collaboration in public services, Sullivan and Skelcher argue that collaboration is the broad church within which contracts, networks and partnerships shelter; 'all collaborative relationships derive from one of three governance forms: contracts, partnerships or networks' (2002: 4). They argue that the partnership mode of governance, though difficult to define, involves collaboration through joint decision-making and production; in contrast, contracts are 'for the most part formal, specific and legally binding agreements between organisations' and networks are 'constituted on the basis of informal relationships regulated by obligations of trust and reciprocity' (4–5). But, in practice, a definition remains a contested issue. Even the related terms suffer from the problem of lack of clarity of definition. For example, Huxham argues that 'collaborative advantage' will be achieved when:

> something unusually creative is produced – perhaps an objective is met – that no organisation could have produced on its own and when each organisation, through the collaboration, is able to achieve its own objectives better than it could alone. In some cases, it should be

> possible to achieve some higher-level ... objectives for society as a whole rather than just for the participating organizations. (1996: 14)

However, Huxham's edited book also provides contrasting definitions of collaborative advantage.

Within this volume a loose definition of 'partnerships' is most commonly adopted; a definition which encompasses other related terms such as 'joint working', 'joint planning', 'networking' and 'collaboration'. In this way the authors reflect the common usage of the term amongst practitioners and policy-makers, where it is used interchangeably with the above terms. A number of articles use many of the terms listed above (Glendinning and Coleman; Snape; Ranade and Hudson). In this way comparatively little effort has been expended by the authors in contributing to further refining the definitions within this field; which in any case appears to be an increasingly fruitless game of diminishing returns.

However, 'joint planning' is the favoured term used by Bridgen, a logical selection given the focus of his paper on the historical sweep of joint working between health and local government in the post-war period. 'Joint planning' was very much the phrase used by contemporaries in the key periods discussed in his article (the 1960s and 1970s) and reflect this period of history when solutions to service problems were viewed as largely in need of strategic joint planning, in retrospect a somewhat one-dimensional approach. The article reviews the development of post-war policy in joint planning between health and social services, with special reference to services for older people. Adopting the traditional concept of the boundary between health and local government (that is, the health and social services interface), Bridgen argues that historical analysis identifies considerable obstacles to joint working. In particular – and rarely recognised before – the broader policy context plays a central role in explaining limited progress. Central government's exhortations to joint planning since the 1960s have been consistently hampered by distrust among local agencies (particularly local authorities) of its more general policy initiatives in this area. And his prognosis for collaboration is bleak; with the necessary conditions for successful joint working (organisational homogeneity, domain consensus and so on) absent both in the past and likely to remain so in the near future.

In their exploration of the conceptual issues underpinning inter-agency collaboration, Ranade and Hudson also reflect on the necessary conditions for collaboration and on the range of barriers frustrating enthusiasts for joint working. They begin by examining the post-1997 policy context for inter-agency working, and argue that a focus on 'co-ordinating partnerships' has given way to a period of 'co-evolving partnerships'. The former aimed to deliver pre-set collective goals in a context of confidence that these were the correct objectives which would produce predictable results. The latter emerged in order to tackle intractable cross-cutting issues in a context where the collective goals are poorly defined and past solutions have failed. Such co-evolving partnerships reflect the shift to more complex and ambitious collaboration in the public sector, requiring new modes of governance. Three such modes of governance are examined in particular – the familiar typology of market, hierarchy and network. Ranade and Hudson argue that these three are best seen as overlain and co-existing. Such a hybrid mode of governance is fraught with paradox, contradiction and tension; contradiction between New Labour's emphasis on partnership while still encouraging competition; and tension between freedom to innovate in inter-agency working and centrally determined systems of performance management and measurement. Central to overcoming these contradictions is a mature understanding of the bases and barriers to collaboration and the strengths and weaknesses of different modes of governance.

The next two contributions to this volume move the reader on from this general conceptual and theoretical debate to discuss the post-1997 policy context from the perspectives of the health services and local government respectively. The first of these 'paired' or 'companion' essays, by Glendinning and Coleman, examines the policy and practice of collaboration between the NHS and local authorities from a health services perspective. In particular, it focuses on collaboration in the area of primary care. Four key themes in the post-1997 policy context are identified which have relevance to this area of collaboration: the move from GP fund-holding to the creation of Primary Care Groups (PCGs) and Primary Care Trusts (PCTs); a shift from treating to preventing illness (reflecting acknowledgement of social, economic and environmental factors to widening inequalities of health); the drive for implementation by central government, involving centrally determined targets and timetables; and, the reorientation of policy away from competition and markets to collaboration and partnerships.

Within this broad policy context, Glendinning and Coleman identify two key issues which are likely to have an impact on the collaborative activities of local government and NHS organisations. First is the intensification – instigated by GP fund-holding – of devolution of responsibility for health care planning and delivery to front-line professionals through the vehicle of PCGs and PCTs. The second issue is the managerial pressures to modernise NHS organisations through performance management, targets, inspection and so on. And there is evidence that the latter is a considerable threat to collaborative adventures since, for example, performance management systems tend to focus more on easier to measure indicators of institutional performance rather than difficult to measure outcomes from inter-agency collaboration. It is not solely the enhanced regulatory regime which is an obstacle, the authors also identify other threats to collaboration, in particular the dominant position of general practitioners (GPs) within PCGs and PCTs. On the positive side, there are factors which the evidence suggests are supporting collaboration; the size, scope, responsibilities and budgets of PCG/Ts may well provide an organisational framework which is more conducive to joint working.

Snape's paper, as a companion article to Coleman and Glendinning's, explores the policy context of joint working from a local government perspective. While giving some attention to changes in the health–social care interface (viewed by Snape as the 'traditional' boundary between health and local government), the author argues that the period since 1997 can be characterised as one in which this traditional boundary has been challenged from the local government perspective by developments such as community governance, new council constitutions and health scrutiny. These developments have provided an opportunity for local authorities to fundamentally rethink their relationship with health. The article finds that some progress has been made but that the traditional boundary casts a long shadow in health–local government relationships.

Complementing the broad policy analysis of Glendinning and Coleman, and Snape, the paper by Cole provides a case study of health–local government partnerships in action by analysing the success and achievements of the Plymouth Health Action Zone. The Health Action Zones – 26 in total – were to provide one of the key arenas for the interplay of the relationship between health and local authorities in the post-1997 policy environment. Although the HAZ programme fell somewhat out of favour with the appointment of Alan Milburn as Secretary of State for Health in 1999, they remain an enduring symbol of New Labour's commitment to area-based partnership initiatives. Cole's article is also interesting since it provides an illustration of the trend towards theory-based models of evaluation for partnership initiatives and, importantly, an assessment of the 'success' of such an approach.

Cole assesses the impact of 37 projects sponsored by the HAZ, exploring the extent to which they used a realistic evaluation/theories of change framework, achieved their project objectives and contributed to the three main objectives of the Plymouth HAZ: developing partnership working; modernising the care system; and, tackling health inequalities. In contrast to some of the more pessimistic views in this field, Cole provides substantive evidence that the Plymouth HAZ made a significant contribution to developing effective partnership working in the city; 'such wide-ranging partnerships appear to be useful as a catalyst to promote joint working between agencies' (115). One element of this success has been identified by Cole as the process of 'cultural convergence'; the reconciling of the medical and social models of health to produce new and integrated models of working.

The seventh and eighth papers in this collection could be viewed as the second set of 'companion' papers, since they share a determination to approach the subject matter of collaboration in non-traditional ways (*non-traditional* for public policy analysis). Hoggett's article deliberately seeks to draw attention to 'overlooked issues' which he views as critical in explaining the continuing difficulty in achieving successful collaboration. The article draws on the sociology of community, psycho-dynamics of inter-group behaviour and theories of identity and difference. Working from these perspectives, the author seeks to explode the myth of the inclusive community, which he argues underpins New Labour thinking. Instead, conflict is both inherent in relations between organisations and necessary for the creation of more enduring relationships. The processes of 'splitting' and 'exclusion' are not only found in geographical communities but also in professional and occupational communities.

Relationships of conflict, hostility, misunderstanding and non-cooperation can be better addressed by understanding concepts such as 'relationships-in-the-mind'. Such concepts are useful in explaining how identities are formed and maintained. Splitting and exclusion can be very useful for groups, in terms of developing a strong sense of 'we-ness' or identity. However, they can significantly undermine initiatives which seek to foster joint working. Hoggett argues that instead of reacting in a way which seeks to suppress these 'emotional' or 'psychological' conflicts, groups must engage in 'conflictual dialogue' which engages fundamentally in what are often dismissed as 'subjective' issues; in other words, groups must tackle openly the misunderstandings created by group identities. Although such an approach is sometimes dismissed as focusing on the 'soft' issues of partnership working, Hoggett believes that down this path lies a greater chance of success in collaboration than some of the more traditional 'hard' approaches, such as structural reorganisation.

Although the focus of Broussine's article is the capacities that local authority chief executives need in order to engage effectively with joined-up working, there are many parallels with Hoggett's paper. As with Hoggett, Broussine explores the 'softer' issues involved in collaboration. His article begins by examining the paradoxical feelings that chief executives can hold about their roles, and moves on to explore the importance of 'emotional' boundaries. Examining concepts such as 'knowing' and 'not knowing', Broussine concludes that there is a premium on the capacities for sense-making through systematic analysis, for maintaining personal perspective and for seeing leadership as synonymous with learning.

It is hoped that this volume provides useful insights and reflections upon the health–local government relationship after six years of New Labour. Although the authors are not united in their views of the future prospects for this pivotal relationship, it is clear from this collection that assessment of the achievements and failures of partnership working benefits from a range of evaluative, theoretical and conceptual approaches, drawing on a mix of disciplines. The work of Broussine and Hoggett clearly points to the value of psycho-social approaches. Undoubtedly, as the practice of partnership working between these two great leviathans of the twenty-first century state continues to evolve, the approaches of academics working in this field will also need to evolve; to find new methods for supporting and analysing this crucial relationship.

NOTES

1. In arguing that these are the key areas of divergence from NPM the authors largely concur with Newman's analysis, which was detailed earlier in the article (2002). However, the authors do not agree with Newman's argument that these two should be joined by a third: 'managers as partners in delivering policy outcomes'.

REFERENCES

Benington, J., 2003, 'From Public Choice to Public Value', IGPM Working Paper, University of Warwick, forthcoming.

Blair, T., 1998, *The Third Way* (London: Fabian Society).

Giddens, A., 1998, *The Third Way: The Renewal of Social Democracy* (Cambridge: Polity Press).

Ferlie, E. and L. Fitzgerald, 2002, 'The Sustainability of the New Public Management in the UK', in McLaughlin *et al.*, 2002.

Ham, C., 1999, 'The Third Way in Health Care Reform – Does the Emperor have Any Clothes?', *Journal of Health Services Research and Policy*, 4/3, pp.168–73.

Hood, C., 1991, 'A Public Management for all Seasons?', *Public Administration*, 61/1, pp.3–19.

Huxham, C. (ed.), 1996, *Creating Collaborative Advantage* (London: Sage).

McLaughlin, K., S.P. Osborne and E. Ferlie (eds.), 2002, *New Public Management: Current Trends and Future Prospects* (London: Routledge).

Moore, M., 1995, *Creating Public Value: Strategic Management in Government* (Harvard University Press: Boston).

Newman, J., 2001, *Modernising Governance: New Labour, Policy and Society* (London: Sage).

Newman, J., 2002, 'The New Public Management, Modernisation and Institutional Change', in McLaughlin *et al.*, 2002.

OECD, 1987, *Managing and Financing Urban Services* (OECD: Paris).

Osborne, D. and T. Gaebler, 1992, *Reinventing Government* (Reading MA: Addison Wesley).

Ranade, W. (ed.) 2001, *Local Governance*, Special Issue on Health and Local Authority Collaboration, 27/4.

Rhodes, R.A.W., 1997, *Understanding Governance: Policy Networks, Governance, Reflexivity and Accountability* (Open University).

Snape, S., 2000, 'Three Years On: Reviewing Local Government Modernisation', *Local Governance*, Special Issue on Local Government Modernisation, 26/3, pp.119–26.

Stoker, G., 2002, 'Life is a Lottery: New Labour's Strategy for the Reform of Devolved Governance', *Public Administration*, 80/3, pp.417–34.

Sullivan, H. and C. Skelcher, 2002, *Working Across Boundaries: Collaboration in Public Services* (Basingstoke: Palgrave Macmillan).

Wistow, G. and B. Hardy, 1991, 'Joint Management in Community Care', *Journal of Management in Medicine*, 5/4.

Joint Planning across the Health/Social Services Boundary since 1946

PAUL BRIDGEN

Exhortations to organisations, professions and other producer interests
to work together more closely and effectively, litter the policy
landscape ... [Y]et the reality is all too often a jumble of services
fractionalised by professional, cultural and organisational boundaries
and by tiers of governance. (Webb, 1991: 229)

This pessimistic assessment of the post-war history of joint working
between public welfare bodies reflects a more general pessimism in the
academic literature about the prospects for inter-organisational
collaboration. Any assumption that organisations working in related fields
will collaborate to enhance the common good, or for altruistic reasons, have
been dismissed as naive. Collaboration involves costs in terms of loss of
control and the investment of scare resources which organisations will
generally seek to avoid (Hudson, 1987). It will thus only occur under certain
conditions. Where there is:

- organisational homogeneity (i.e. structural, cultural similarity);
- domain consensus (i.e. agreement on what each organisation will and
  will not do);
- an awareness within organisations of their interdependence (i.e. network
  awareness);
- benefit to be gained for both sides;
- an absence of alternative organisations with which to collaborate.

If these conditions are not present an outside agency (i.e. an executive body
or legislative body) may be required to encourage organisations to co-
operate by incentives or direction.

In no area has the disjunction between the exhortation and
implementation of joint working been greater than in proposals for the joint
planning of health and social services for older people. The last 40 years has
seen repeated policy initiatives proposed to encourage collaboration in this
area, but, as many commentators have suggested, it is in this policy field
that progress has been most limited (e.g. Booth, 1981; Wistow *et al.*, 1990).

This article will focus on this most problematic area for joint working. It will review the development of post-war policy in this area and outline the main obstacles that have been identified as inhibitors of progress. In this regard, it will concentrate on the nature of the organisations on the two sides of the health/social services boundary and debates about the respective responsibilities of these organisations.[1] However, it will also suggest that, if the problems encountered with joint planning are to be properly understood, the broader policy context within which these initiatives took place must be investigated. In this regard, previous reviews of developments in this area have sometimes tended to concentrate on the relationship between the two sides of the health/social services boundary, with the role of central government, its motives for seeking to encourage joint working and the effect this had on the joint planning process treated as largely unproblematic (e.g. Nocon, 1994).[2] What this article will suggest, in contrast, is that central government's attempts to encourage joint planning since the 1960s have repeatedly been hampered by distrust among local agencies of its more general policy intentions in this area. In this regard, local authorities, in particular, have regarded joint planning as part of a broader process, whereby the responsibility for long-term care has gradually been passed from hospitals to them, with inadequate financial compensation.

In order to investigate these issues in more detail it is first necessary to have a full sense of the multi-dimensional nature of the boundary between health and social services; the reasons for its persistence; and the major issues that have arisen as a result. This is the purpose of the next section. The article will then consider the joint planning initiatives of the 1960s and 1970s, before, in the final section, a cautious attempt is made to assess recent joint planning developments over the past 15 years.

THE BOUNDARY BETWEEN HEALTH AND SOCIAL SERVICES, 1946–97

The boundary between health and social services has been a permanent feature of post-war British welfare provision. It came into existence as part of the establishment of the NHS in 1946. The then minister of health Aneurin Bevan's decision to nationalise the hospital service meant that local authorities lost all their pre-war responsibilities for secondary care.[3] They were left with responsibility for providing residential accommodation under part III of the 1948 National Assistance Act, together with a range of domiciliary services, including home nursing and home helps.

There were mixed opinions among health officials at the time about the potential for problems created by this division of functions. Some, in the optimistic atmosphere of the early NHS years and influenced by a strong belief in the public service ethic (Webb, 1991), argued that:

[because] the hospital system with which local authorities will be in contact will be a government system ... although occasions for friction will arise they will not be pursued or perpetrated as is often the case at present ... It seems probable that the mere existence of these two sets of services side by side will produce day by day co-operation both in minor and major matters, and through that association will inevitably come the integration which is desired (PRO, MH 80/33).

Other officials, however, were less sanguine and believed the boundary would ultimately prove unsustainable. One NHS official, for example, wrote in September 1949: 'It would seem to be a corollary of the scheme that we should later, if not sooner, take over all the personal health services' (PRO, MH 80/34). This, in fact did occur, but not until 1974, when as part of a thoroughgoing reorganisation process, district nursing and health visiting were transferred from local authority control to the NHS. This did not remove the boundary, but made the division between health and social service functions more definite (Brown, 1979).

The option of removing the boundary completely either by transferring all social services to the NHS, or through the creation of the local authority health service, has been regularly debated, but has never been proposed by government (Webster, 1988). The medical profession has strongly resisted a locally run health service and successfully managed to keep this option off the agenda.[4] However, the local government and social work lobby, in combination, has managed to prevent an NHS takeover of social service functions.

Despite being repeatedly emphasised as a policy problem since 1946, therefore, the boundary has survived. It is a boundary that is made up of a number of different dimensions. The administrative division of health and social services has meant that the governance of the two services has differed in important ways. They differ, for example, in their planning cycles, budgetary procedures and accountability systems (Rogers, 1979). The boundary also consists of a financial division. Thus, while health authorities are funded directly from central taxation, local authorities receive some of their money (approximately 80 per cent by the mid-1990s) from central taxation in the form of a grant, which is not ring-fenced, and raise the rest themselves from a local property-based tax. There is also a professional division at the boundary. The NHS has since its creation been dominated by the medical profession. Social services, in contrast, have been dominated, particularly since the early 1960s, by the social work profession who have been suspicious of the 'medical model' and sought to resist medical domination of their work.

Disputes about the respective responsibilities of health and local authorities have been at the heart of debates about the boundary. The question of responsibilities was bound to be problematic, given the complexity and variability of the needs of the older people using health and social services, and any definition of respective responsibilities was only ever likely to provide a general guide. However, argument about this issue has been made more intense by the suspicion among local authorities that they have been expected to take on greater care responsibilities. In this regard, responsibility for the continuing care of older people, not requiring medical intervention, but too ill to remain at home, has been the central issue. In 1946, health officials decided that local authorities should be responsible for those in 'need of care and attention, [but] not ... constant medical and nursing attention', with hospitals taking responsibility for 'those in need of constant medical and nursing attention and those who are incapacitated by mental disorder' (PRO, MH80/47). This definition, it was strongly intimated by health officials at the time, meant that hospitals would be responsible for older people requiring continuing care. It remained substantially unchanged for the next 50 years (Bridgen and Lewis, 2000), but, as will be seen, local authorities have repeatedly complained that it was being ignored both by hospitals and central government.

This dispute about respective responsibilities has been made more problematic by the financial and professional aspects of the boundary. Differing funding arrangements, together with the fact that resources have often been severely limited, has made it tempting for both local authorities and health authorities to minimise their responsibilities (Glennerster, 1983). Professional considerations have also encouraged this phenomenon. Hall and Bytheway have suggested, for example, that hospital doctors have sought to limit the definition of health care in line with the prevailing 'acute ideology' in medicine, and have thus tried to restrict entry to hospitals by controlling assessments of patients' needs (1991; see also Martin, 1995).

Thus, some of the basic elements required, according to the theoretical literature, for collaboration to be successful have always been absent between the two sides of the health/social services divide. Administrative, financial and professional differences mean the bodies on the two sides of the boundary have always lacked organisational homogeneity; and the constant debate about respective responsibilities indicates the persistent absence of domain consensus.

As the review of the literature that follows will show, the lack of these elements has featured heavily in assessments of joint planning. However, what will also be shown is that the overall policy context within which joint planning was proposed, and the perception of this policy context by those who were asked to engage in this process, particularly local authorities, has made joint planning even more problematic.

JOINT PLANNING IN THE 1950s/60s

Joint planning, as opposed to other forms of joint working, was not explicitly encouraged between the health and social services until the early 1960s. Problems had been apparent at the boundary between health and social care before this time. Indeed, complaints about responsibility shifting from both sides began almost as soon as the new system began to operate (PRO, MH 99/116). However, up to the mid-1950s, central government's response was to adopt a position of neutrality and blame the problems on inadequate resources on both sides of the boundary, a situation which would only be addressed once the difficult financial conditions of the early post-war period had eased. In the meantime, the two sides were encouraged to collaborate on operational matters to ensure service-users did not suffer. 'The only thing necessary was goodwill ... to make sure that everybody was catered for', Ministry officials insisted (PRO, MH 130/266).

Joint planning emerged in the early 1960s as a method for achieving a specific policy goal. It was intended to facilitate a shift in the locus of care for the elderly from hospitals to the home. The provenance of this policy is well known. It emerged from the mid-1950s as part of the development of ideas about community care and geriatric medicine, which suggested that many elderly people who currently received long-term care (of questionable quality) in hospital beds, could, with an active approach to their treatment, be rehabilitated and returned home (Wilkin et al., 1986; and Brocklehurst, 1977). This would not involve a change in the care responsibilities of hospitals and local authorities, it was argued, because, while a greater number of older people would be discharged from hospital, they would only require the types of services provided by local authorities (Bridgen and Lewis, 2000). The treatment they received in hospital would be improved making them fit to return to the community.

In fact, while these ideas about geriatric care represented an important advance on pre-war medical treatment of older people (Webster, 1991), their potential was considerably over-estimated in government (Bridgen and Lewis, 2000; and Bridgen, 2001). Health officials, increasingly anxious about the cost of the hospital service and under pressure from hospital doctors anxious to reduce the 'burden' imposed by older people on hospital care, substantially exaggerated the extent to which they would reduce the number of older people requiring long-term hospital care. Some recognised that in reality any accelerated discharge of older people from hospital would involve an increase in local authority care responsibilities, but this was not made explicit (PRO, MH 99/163).

The purpose of the 1962 hospital plan and 1963 local health and welfare plan was to entrench this policy in the future development of health and social services (*A Hospital Plan for England and Wales*, Cmnd. 1604, 1962; *Health and Welfare: the Development of Community Care*, Cmnd. 1973, 1963). Thus, while the former envisaged the ten-year development of a £500 million network of new hospitals, this only involved an increase in geriatric beds in line with the projected growth in the number of elderly people (Bridgen and Lowe, 1998). Increasingly, the assumption among some health officials was that long-term care for the elderly would become a non-hospital function. To this end, local authorities were asked to collaborate with their local hospitals to plan the expansion of domiciliary services to meet the needs of the greater number of discharged older patients (PRO MH134/42). They were promised an increase in resources of 3.75 per cent a year for five years to do so.

As a number of commentators have suggested, this first experiment in joint planning was almost entirely unsuccessful. A 1969 survey of local authorities' implementation of the local health and welfare plan, for example, found that while 'plans were sometimes ... discussed with other bodies, such as hospitals ... the tendency was to plan each service separately, and without allowance for the possibility of substitution of one service or group of services for another' (Sumner and Smith, 1969: 209). Moreover, rather than concentrating on domiciliary care as the Ministry had hoped, the major area of expansion proposed by the local authorities was in residential provision (*Health and Welfare*: paras.54–60).[5]

It is easy enough in hindsight to identify, on the basis of the theoretical insights about inter-organisational collaboration outlined above, problems with the joint planning initiative of the early 1960s.[6] Central government was hoping for collaboration between organisations with significant structural and cultural differences, which had been for the previous decade in almost constant dispute about their respective responsibilities. To this end, its only intervention was in the form of exhortation by circulars. The two sides could be relied upon, central government believed, to overcome the problems caused by the boundary out of a concern for the public good.

However, what also needs to be emphasised in any assessment of the plans of the early 1960s is the lack of consensus that existed about the policy goal joint planning was designed to achieve, and the way this impinged on the exercise. Local authorities, in particular, questioned the whole basis on which the planning process was being encouraged by central government. They believed the underlying objectives of the plans was to reduce the responsibilities of hospitals for geriatric care at the expense of local authorities, despite denials by the Ministry (PRO MH134/41). The emphasis placed by the ministry on domiciliary care increased suspicions in this regard. Local authorities feared that an expansion in domiciliary services might encourage hospitals to discharge elderly people with greater degrees of infirmity more quickly (or refuse them admission for longer) in the knowledge that local authorities would be less able to refuse responsibility for their care. Whereas local authorities had some means of controlling the flow between hospitals and their residential accommodation, this was less true with regard to the flow between hospitals and domiciliary services (Bridgen and Lewis, 2000).[7] Given these concerns about the underlying aims of the plan, local authorities thus made clear that they would only co-operate with the joint planning exercise if far better financial guarantees were made. They warned the ministry of the 'need for increased grant to take account of the expanding services of local authorities ... particularly in relation to some services (e.g. home helps) where [they] were more and more undertaking functions hitherto undertaken by the hospital authorities' (Means and Smith, 1985: 266).

Thus, central government, in its facilitation of joint planning between health and social services, was not regarded as neutral in the dispute over responsibilities, but an interested party, sympathetic to the views of the health authorities. As has been seen, local authorities had some justification for this belief. Thus, while structural problems and pre-existing disputes about responsibilities made joint planning between health and social services, in any case, extremely problematic, the policy context in which the planning process of the early 1960s was proposed only served to exacerbate these difficulties. The government's motives in seeking to encourage joint planning were questioned, with the consequence that levels of distrust rose, particularly among local authorities.

THE FAILURE OF VOLUNTARY CO-OPERATION

The failure of the planning exercise of the early 1960s convinced commentators and policy-makers that exhortation by itself was unlikely to lead to joint planning. As the Seebohm Report observed, for example:

> [n]either the evidence we have received nor the visits and discussions we have had convince us that any of [the] means for securing co-ordinated action work satisfactorily. Although the success achieved obviously varies in different areas, overall the impression is of very limited success despite the expenditure of much time and energy. (*Report of the Committee on Local Authority and Allied Personal Social Services*, Cmnd 3703: para.70)

The Report pinpointed some of the structural explanations for the failure of voluntary collaborative planning which were later to prove influential. The problem was, it explained, that 'the financial interests and regulations of local authorities and (the hospital service) do not always coincide' (para.69). The relationship between the local authority social services and the NHS thus needed to undergo a 'reconstruction'. 'There is need', the Report added, 'for imaginative ideas for trying new approaches and a refusal to be satisfied with any particular method merely because it has always been used in the past' (para.307).

This evidence, together with the realisation that the new structural settlement established by the 1974 reorganisation would tighten the division between the two sides, convinced DHSS officials that a more active policy had to be introduced to improve the situation. The 'coterminosity' of the boundaries between health and local authorities, established as part of the 1974 reorganisation, was held to be insufficient (DHSS, 1971a). A new statutory machinery for collaboration was recommended. Thus it was proposed that:

1. Area health authorities and local authorities should be required to set up joint consultative committees (JCCs), comprising members from the two sets of authorities.
2. Health and local authorities should have the power to provide each other with resources and make staff available for the use of the other authority (Glennerster, 1983: 18).

In addition, in 1976 joint care planning teams (JCPTs) made up of officers were established to assist the joint planning process (DHSS, 1976a); and joint finance was introduced, by which health authorities were granted funds to finance the development of services by local authorities (DHSS, 1977). This exercise in statutory joint planning, health and local authorities were told, should be genuinely collaborative and not merely involve 'the joint consideration of plans that had been prepared separately' (DHSS, 1973: para.2.13). It was hoped that agreement would be reached on a common approach to needs assessment; and the desirable balance of care between, and range of services offered by, both sides.

ASSESSING 1970s JOINT PLANNING

Despite these initiatives, assessments of joint planning established in the 1970s have generally been equally as negative as those undertaken a decade earlier. In 1984, a DHSS working group on joint planning reported that:

> joint planning showed promise in some areas but over the country as a whole these services had generally not developed as they should have done ... [T]here was a widespread sense of frustration that more had not been achieved ... While there is virtually unanimous intellectual assent to the importance of getting health and local

authorities and voluntary organisations to work together, in practice progress has been disappointing. (DHSS, 1984: i)

This conclusion was supported by Booth in his case study of joint planning during the mid-1970s in Calderdale. He found that:

> there was a deep-rooted and sincere conviction among all participants from both sides of the JCPT that the main aim of developing a joint strategic approach to the planning of the health and personal social services is a desirable objective. There was also a considerable degree of unanimity about the potential benefits of such collaboration. However, participants were a great deal more cautious over whether the aim of forging partnership in planning matters of common concern was a realistic and attainable one. (Booth, 1981: 41)

In only a very few areas were joint care strategies agreed, and where they were, most were not implemented. JCCs, in particular, had quickly become regarded merely as 'talking shops' and 'rubber stamps' (Glennerster, 1983).

Wistow, however, was less pessimistic (1988). Certainly, joint planning was not a success judged by the goals that were set for it, but these were 'over-ambitious'. In fact, in comparison with the 1960s exercise important progress was made. Planning moved from being entirely separate to being parallel and mutually sensitive. Inter-organisational relationships became much closer and joint working was pushed higher up the agendas of both authorities. Moreover, at the operational level significant progress was made.

Despite this more optimistic assessment, the failure of joint planning to achieve as much as had been hoped led commentators to analyse more closely the structural, procedural and professional impediments it faced (Glennerster, 1983; and Wistow et al., 1990). The differences in the funding structure, planning cycle and decision-making process of the two authorities were identified as major problems. Differences in the perspective of the various professional groups operating within the two authorities had also created problems. These had been made worse by the fact that the introduction of joint planning had coincided with the setting up of the new post-Seebohm social services departments, in which a newly established and self-confident social work profession was seeking to assert its independence.

It was thus concluded that the mechanisms put in place in 1974 and 1976 had failed to overcome these obstacles. Webster, for example, dismissed the new structures as 'innocuous' (1988; see also Glennerester, 1983; Webb and Wistow, 1987; and Klein, 1989). It was far from clear how joint planning was meant to be achieved, even after more detailed advice about the structure of the new bodies was issued in DHSS circulars of 1976 and 1977 (DHSS, 1976a; and DHSS, 1977). What was clear, however, was that the new structures had no executive functions (DHSS, 1976a).[8] Similarly, while joint finance had encouraged greater interest in joint planning, particularly in the local authorities, little of it had been used to fund new collaborative ventures (Glennerster, 1983; Wistow, 1990)

The limited nature of the 1970s joint planning reform was held to reflect the fact that ultimately the Department still believed that 'goodwill' between the two parties was the best guarantee of co-operation, a view that the 1973 working party on collaboration, which had recommended the establishment of the new bodies, seemed to support (DHSS, 1973).

However, while structural problems were the main focus of attention in the mid-1980s, they were not the only obstacles to joint planning. There is also strong evidence to suggest that central government's failure to address some of the concerns about its broader policy framework also played a major part in undermining the initiative in the 1970s/80s, as it had done in the 1960s. In this regard, the policy goal for joint planning remained the same: to shift the focus of care for the elderly and other vulnerable 'priority' groups from hospitals to local authorities. Statutory joint planning was thus one of a series of initiatives launched between 1972 and 1977 which sought to address the problems encountered during the 1960s in achieving this policy goal. To meet local authorities' previous concerns about resources, for example, they were promised a sizeable increase in expenditure, including a six per cent annual rise in investment on home nursing and health visitors (DHSS, 1976b).[9] The DHSS also took a more directive approach with regard to the nature of local authority plans, with departmental guidelines established on the basis of research undertaken by or for the DHSS.

However, with respect to the question of responsibilities there was no change in health officials' approach. They continued to deny that the policy of shifting the balance of care entailed a reduction in the non-acute role of the hospitals, despite evidence to the contrary. In this regard, government documents continued to display an ambivalence about the hospitals' role in long-term care of the elderly. 'Bed-blocking', for example, was blamed entirely on the failure of local authorities to provide 'sufficient domiciliary and residential care' (DHSS, 1976b: para.5.10). Evidence that it was also a result of the failure of hospitals to take responsibility for long-term patients was ignored (DHSS, 1971b; DHSS, 1972). Moreover, repeated emphasis was given to the benefits of reducing the average length of hospital stays (DHSS, 1976b: para.4.22).

This ambivalence at central government level about the hospitals' role in long-term care appears to have fed through to the joint planning process at the local level. As Booth found in his case study of Calderdale, the health authority side regarded joint planning quite simply as a method for ensuring that the local authority side 'accept[ed] its share of the responsibility for the care of the elderly' (1981: 35). The result was that the emphasis of the process was 'rather pointedly on getting the local authority to give greater priority to services for the elderly and on giving doctors a greater say in who use[d] them' (1981: 37). The focus of collaboration was slanted in favour of the health authority's interests. This immediately provoked a negative response from the local authority, which claimed that its level of provision for the elderly was above DHSS guidelines. Despite the setting up of a special sub-committee to discuss these issues, the problems proved largely irresolvable. Continued differences over responsibilities and priorities helped cause the whole process to become 'stuck in a rut' (1981: 224).

JOINT PLANNING, 1991–2001

This brief history of the first 25 years of joint planning has shown that while organisational differences and an absence of domain consensus made collaboration difficult, these difficulties were greatly exacerbated by the broader policy context in which joint planning initiatives were tried. For local authorities, in particular, joint planning was seen as part of a process, encouraged by central government, whereby their care responsibilities were surreptitiously increased without adequate financial compensation. This suspicion greatly complicated their discussions with health authorities.

In the last 15 years, the flaws in the broader policy framework of community care have begun to receive greater attention. The 1986 Audit Commission report, *Making a Reality of Community Care*, for example, emphasised central government's failure to guarantee local authorities the resources to develop community care and the 'organizational fragmentation and confusion in responsibilities at all levels'. It also proposed the pooling of elderly care budgets between health and local authorities with the aim of reducing the financial incentives for responsibility shifting. As Wistow has suggested, the Commission, in raising doubts about broader policy, helped shift the emphasis with respect to community care 'from the failure of local agencies to collaborate effectively to the responsibility of central government for this failure' (Wistow, 1988: 74).

However, the response of the Conservative government of the late 1980s and early 1990s to these criticisms was only partial. While, for example, greater resources were transferred to local authorities to develop community services in the early 1990s, these were not permanently ring-fenced as the Audit Commission and the government's own Griffiths report had recommended (DH, 1988). The more detailed recommendations made by the Audit Commission with respect to joint working were ignored.

Moreover, on the question of responsibilities, the Audit Commission itself had only dealt with one part of the issue. It focused on 'confused responsibilities' at the community service level and did not address the broader question of hospitals' responsibilities for long-term care. Central government was again let off the hook with regard to the implications of community care for the scope of the NHS. Health officials continued to insist in the early 1990s that 'the key functions and responsibilities of the health service ... remain essentially unaltered' (DH, 1989: para.4.2).

Thus, the broader policy problems which had greatly complicated previous joint planning efforts were only partially addressed. Joint planning continued to be promoted, however, albeit that the importance of JCCs and JCPTs was increasingly de-emphasised (DH, 1989: para.6.12). In the development of new community care plans, local authorities were 'expected to work closely with relevant health authorities in planning community care services' (DH, 1990: 38). Why this should be any more achievable in the early 1990s, given that many of the problems that had prevented it occurring previously remained, was not made clear. Predictably, in these circumstances, assessments of the community care plans of the early 1990s echoed judgements of previous joint planning initiatives (e.g. Salter and Salter, 1993).

Despite this unpromising history, the concept of joint working has been enthusiastically re-launched by New Labour since 1997 (e.g. DH, 1998). The last five years have seen the acceptance – and almost immediate extension – of greater financial flexibilities at the boundary, including pooled budgets; the introduction of a new duty of partnership on health and local authorities; and a renewed commitment to joint planning, in the shape of health improvement plans (HiMPs) – and, with respect to the development of services for older people and other particularly vulnerable groups, joint investment plans (JIPs). These initiatives have been backed up by the threat that central government might impose an integrated 'care trust' on local areas where collaboration does not occur (Lewis, 2001).[10]

But are these new initiatives likely to be any more successful in encouraging joint planning than those of the previous 40 years? In answering this question, caution is required. History carries no prescriptive power. Yet, some observations are still possible.

In this regard, there are a few minor reasons to be optimistic. Some policy learning does appear to have taken place. There does now seem to be an acceptance by central government of the extent of the structural and cultural obstacles in the way of joint planning and the need for policy interventions more sophisticated than exhortation. In this regard, the issue of respective responsibilities, which has plagued joint planning initiatives in the past, has been addressed more directly in the last four years than at any other time during the previous 40. The introduction of pooled budgets, together with the decision (in partial response to the recommendations of the Royal Commission on Long-Term Care) to make 'registered nursing' an NHS responsibility regardless of institutional setting, should both, in theory, reduce the incentives on the two sides of the boundary to responsibility shift.11 These changes should also help reduce the salience of the dispute about long-term care, a process that is further assisted by the Department of Health's recent recognition that the nature of hospitals' responsibilities in this area has changed (DH, 2001).

Yet many problems remain in this area and others, and if this brief survey of the history of joint planning of services for older people shows nothing else, it does reveal the entrenched nature of the obstacles in the way of a genuinely collaborative approach to joint working. Progress there has been over the last 40 years, but it has been slow and incremental. There seems little reason to believe that the pace of developments in the future will be very much different.

ACKNOWLEDGEMENT

The author would like to acknowledge the assistance of Jane Lewis in writing this article. The research on which it is based was funded by Nuffield Provincial Hospitals Trust.

NOTES

1. Network awareness has not been a problem with respect to the boundary between health and social service, nor do the two sides have any alternative organisations with which to collaborate
2. However, Wistow (1988) does mention the importance of this broader context in his assessment of the prospects for joint planning in the 1990s.
3. Nationalisation occurred in the hope that a hospital service with nationally uniform standards would result.
4. There have also been financial and accountability difficulties with such a proposal given the limited tax base of local government.
5. This concentration on residential provision reflected the fact that most local authorities had long waiting lists for their homes and that many older people remained housed in pre-war Poor Law buildings, despite a 1940s commitment to abolish this form of provision. *Local Health and Welfare*, paras.54–60.
6. Most of the theoretical literature was written after these problems occurred.
7. This situation had become apparent during the course of the Ministry of Health's *Survey of Services Available to the Chronic Sick and Elderly, 1954–5*, which found that a 'common criticism' from home nurses was that hospitals discharged elderly patients 'prematurely' into their care.
8. The DHSS stated categorically that 'the role of JCPTs is advisory not executive'.
9. However, this spending target was quickly jettisoned as part of the response to the 1976 economic crisis.
10. The power to impose Care Trusts was watered down in the final legislation, but it remains an option central government might consider in future.

11. Clearly, this is even more the case with regard to Scotland, where the Scottish Executive has decided, in line with the Royal Commission's recommendations, to make 'personal care' free.

REFERENCES

A Hospital Plan for England and Wales, 1962, Cmnd. 1604 (London: HMSO).

Audit Commission, 1986, *Making a Reality of Community Care* (London: HMSO).

Booth, T.A., 1981, 'Collaboration between Health and Social Services: Part II', *Policy and Politics*, 9/1, pp.23–49.

Booth, T.A., 1981, 'Collaboration between Health and Social Services: Part II', *Policy and Politics*, 9/2, pp.205–26.

Bridgen, P. and R. Lowe, 1998, *Welfare Policy under the Conservatives 1951–1964* (London: PRO).

Bridgen, P. and J. Lewis, 1999, *Elderly People and the Boundary between Health and Social Care 1946–91: Whose Responsibility?* (London: Nuffield Trust).

Bridgen, P., 2001, 'Hospitals, Geriatric Medicine and the Long-term Care of Elderly People 1946–1976', *Social History of Medicine*, 14/3, pp.507–23.

Brown, R.G.S., 1979, *Reorganising the National Health Service* (Oxford: Blackwell).

Brocklehurst, J.C., 1983, *The Textbook of Geriatric Medicine* (Edinburgh: Churchill Livingstone).

DH, 1988, *Community Care: An Agenda for Action* (London: DHSS).

DH, 1989, *Caring for People*, Cmnd.849 (London: HMSO).

DH, 1990, *Community Care in the Next Decade and Beyond: Policy guidance* (London: HMSO).

DH, 1998, *Partnership in Action (New Opportunities for Joint Working between Health and Social Services)* (London: DH).

DH, 2001, 'Continuing Care: NHS and Local Council's responsibilities', Circular HSC 2001/015.

DHSS, 1971a, *National Health Service Reorganisation: Consultative Document* (London: DHSS).

DHSS, 1971b, *The Report of the Hospital Advisory Service* (London: DHSS).

DHSS, 1972, *The Report of the Hospital Advisory Service* (London: DHSS).

DHSS, 1973, *A Report from the Working Party on Collaboration on its Activities to the end of 1972* (London: HMSO).

DHSS, 1976a, 'Joint Care Planning: Health and Local Authorities', Circular HC(76)18 (London: DHSS).

DHSS, 1976b, *Priorities for Health and Personal Social Services in England: A Consultative Document* (London: DHSS).

DHSS, 1977, 'Joint Care Planning: Health and Local Authorities', Circular HC(77)17 (London: DHSS).

DHSS, 1984, *Progress in Partnership: Report of the Working Group on Joint Planning* (London: DHSS).

DHSS, 1989, *Caring for People*, Cmnd. 849 (London: HMSO).

Hall, D. and B. Bytheway, 1982, 'The Blocked Bed: Definition of a Problem', *Social Science and Medicine*, 16, pp.1985–91.

Glennerster, H. (with N. Korman and F. Marsden-Wilson), 1983, *Planning for Priority Groups* (Oxford: Martin Robertson).

Health and Welfare: the Development of Community Care, 1963, Cmnd. 1973 (London: HMSO).

Hudson, B., 1987, 'Collaboration in Social Welfare: A Framework for Analysis', *Policy and Politics*, 15/3, pp.175–82.

Jefferys, M., 1977, 'The Elderly in the United Kingdom', in A.N. Exton-Smith and J.G. Evans (eds.), *Care of the Elderly: Meeting the Challenge of Dependency* (London: Academic Press).

Klein, R., 1989, *The Politics of the National Health Service* (London: Longman).

Lewis, J., 2001, 'Older People and the Health–Social Care Boundary in the UK: Half a Century of Hidden Policy Conflict', *Social Policy and Administration*, 35/4, pp.343–59.

Martin, M., 1995, 'Medical Knowledge and Medical Practice: Geriatric Medicine in the 1950s', *Social History of Medicine*, 7/3.

Means, R. and R. Smith, 1985, *The Development of Welfare Services for the Elderly* (London: Croom Helm).

Ministry of Health, 1957, *Survey of Services available to the Chronic Sick and Elderly, 1954–5* (London: HMSO).

Nocon, A., 1994, *Collaboration in Community Care in the 1990s* (Sunderland: Business Education Publishers Limited).

Public Record Office, Kew (henceforward PRO), MH 80/33, Briefing memorandum, 28 Feb. 1946.

PRO, MH 80/34, official memorandum, Sept. 1949.

PRO MH 80/47, undated memorandum on the abolition of the Poor Law.

PRO, MH 99/116, letter by Godber to HMCs and RHBs, 19 Jan. 1952.

PRO, MH 99/163, Halliday memorandum, 3 Nov. 1961.

PRO, MH 130/266, Pater notes on memorandum, 15 Nov. 1952.

PRO MH 134/41, County Council Association to Dodds, 12 Oct. 1961.

PRO MH134/42, 'Long Term Plan for Development of Local Authority Health and Welfare Services: Notes for Use in Discussions with Authorities', 2 April 1962.

Report of the Committee on Local Authority and Allied Personal Social Services, 1968, Cmnd. 3703 (London: HMSO).

Rogers, S., 1979, 'Collaboration between Health and Local Authorities: Some Problems and Some Developments', in C. Ham and R. Smith (eds.), *Policies for the Elderly* (Bristol: School for Advanced Urban Studies).

Salter, B. and C. Slater, 1993, 'Theatre of the Absurd', *Health Service Journal*, 11 Nov.

Sumner, G. and R. Smith, 1969, *Planning Local Authority Services for the Elderly* (London: Allen and Unwin).

Webb, A. and G. Wistow, 1987, *Social Work, Social Care and Social Planning: Personal Social Services Since Seebohm* (Harlow: Longman).

Webb, A., 1991, 'Coordination: A Problem in Public Sector Management', *Policy and Politics*, 19/4, pp.229–41.

Webster, C., 1988, *The Health Services since the War*, Vol.1 (London: HMSO).

Webster, C., 1991, 'The Elderly and the Early National Health Service', in M. Pelling, and R.M. Smith (eds.), *Life, Death and the Elderly* (London: Routledge).

Wilkin, D. and B. Hughes, 1986, 'The Elderly and the Health Services', in C. Phillipson and A. Walker (eds.), *Ageing and Social Policy* (Aldershot: Gower).

Wistow, G., 1988, 'Health and Local Authority Collaboration: Lessons and Prospects', in G. Wistow and T. Brooks (eds.), *Joint Management and Joint Planning* (London: Royal Institute of Public Administration).

Wistow, G., B. Hardy and A. Turrell, 1990, *Collaboration Under Financial Constraint: Health Authorities Spending on Joint Finance* (Aldershot: Avebury).

Conceptual Issues in Inter-Agency Collaboration

WENDY RANADE and BOB HUDSON

The rhetoric of 'partnership' has become the *sine qua non* of New Labour's approach to governance in health, social care and regeneration. 'Command and control' systems associated with Old Labour were deemed to be outmoded, while market-type solutions – the hallmark of 'New Right' approaches in the 1990s – were condemned on ideological and practical grounds. Partnership working, hitherto a fringe player in British social policy, was the new 'Third Way' and both Labour governments have produced a stream of legislation, policy guidance and 'best practice' alongside some additional funding, to develop this approach. Much of the initial focus was upon the so-called 'Berlin Wall' between the NHS and social services, but the strategy has extended well beyond this intersection to reflect the application of the model to more complex 'wicked' issues requiring a holistic, multi-faceted approach. This has especially been the case with area-based regeneration initiatives such as Sure Start (pre-school development), Action zones for Education, Employment and Health, New Deal for Communities, Neighbourhood Renewal, Community Safety and others. The sheer proliferation of initiatives has required new strategic co-ordinating partnerships (Local Strategic Partnerships) which are the vehicles for community planning on a city, county or district scale.

Partnerships between statutory, voluntary and private organisations are clearly not new, but are now expected to contain a wider range of stakeholders, and in particular be more inclusive of local communities. In part this reflects another strand of government policy which involves strengthening the 'community governance' role of local authorities (DETR, 1998) and creating new opportunities for people to be involved in decisions which affect them. The new partnerships also have more ambitious aims and objectives. Many of the older forms of inter-agency collaboration – for example Joint Consultative Committees between the health service and social service departments or inter-agency arrangements for child protection – were concerned with co-ordination in the sense Pratt *et al.* (1999) define it. The goals are collective, and the behaviour necessary to achieve them is relatively known and predictable.

Co-ordinating partnerships come together with the intention of delivering pre-set objectives. There is confidence that the objectives are the right ones, knowable from past patterns. The driving force may be a desire to reduce duplication, to add value, by pooling resources or to fit the parts better together. This is the jigsaw model, where, as long as everyone shares the same picture, they can in time see how all their separate pieces fit together. (10)

Many of the new partnerships however were formed to tackle intractable issues cutting across social, economic and environmental categories – the regeneration of the inner cities, educational underachievement, inequalities in health. In government documents there was a strong emphasis on 'joined up' thinking and action, which would bring the 'whole system' to bear on issues which had defeated every government in the past. In this type of collaboration, which Pratt *et al.* call 'co-evolving partnerships', collective goals are much less well defined than the objectives of co-ordination, the time frame is long and the behaviour required to achieve solutions much less knowable. By definition old ways of working have not worked – that is why these problems are intractable. The partners are attempting to co-design something new together for a shared purpose, based on an understanding of the 'whole system' and the interdependence of its parts. Theoretically the notion of co-evolution is based on the way all members of an ecological system evolve together and the way in which the fate of each individual depends on the fate of the eco-system (Capra, 1997; Pratt *et al.*, 1999). Clearly this kind of collaboration requires even more commitment from partner agencies and individuals than co-ordinating partnerships, as Pratt's list of necessary conditions suggests (see Figure 1). It also requires greater realism and sophistication about the constraints and blockages, and how they might be overcome.

FIGURE 1
NECESSARY CONDITIONS FOR SUCCESS IN CO-EVOLVING PARTNERSHIPS

Building relationships: people need time to explore purpose.
Changing mental maps: so that people see themselves as part of a whole and stop shifting blame to other parts of the system.
Diversity: sufficient mix of people from different levels and organisations to enable new possibilities to emerge.
Expectations: that change can be fuelled by passion and energy, not just money and that common purpose is the source of coherence.
Iteration: people need to be able to try and try again.
Leadership: facilitating common ownership and responsibility for the behaviour of the 'whole' as well as one's own individual behaviour.
Future: incentives which enlarge future possibilities and enable people to see their future as linked.

Source: Adapted from Pratt *et al.*, 1999.

As a contribution, this article explores some of the conceptual issues underpinning inter-agency collaboration which help to clarify the context within which the new partnership rhetoric is embedded, and the implications of this for collaboration in practice. The article draws on research and theory from a variety of perspectives, including a number of recent papers and reports by the authors (Hudson *et al.*, 2001; Ranade, 1998; 2000).

PARTNERSHIPS AND MODES OF GOVERNANCE

Social science literature identifies three 'pure' routes to social co-ordination or governance – hierarchy, markets and networks (Frances *et al.*, 1991) – and these provide a useful starting point for analysing the recent history of public service delivery and hence the context within which current collaborations take place. The main characteristics of the three as 'ideal types' are set out in Figure 2.

Up to the end of the 1970s hierarchy was the dominant route to the delivery of public services, with intra-agency co-ordination achieved through the distinctive features of bureaucracy – vertical integration, clearly

FIGURE 2
MODES OF GOVERNANCE – MARKETS HIERARCHIES AND NETWORKS

Key Features	Markets	Hierarchies	Networks
Normative basis strengths	Contract/property rights	Employment relationship	Complementary strengths
Means of communication	Prices	Routines	Relational
Means of conflict reputational concerns	Haggling – resort to law	Administrative fiat – supervision	Norm of reciprocity/ reputational concerns
Degree of flexibility	High	Low	Medium
Amount of commitment among the parties	Low	Medium	High
Tone or climate	Precision and/or Suspicion	Formal, bureaucratic	High, open-ended, mutual benefits
Actor preferences or choices	Independent	Dependent	Interdependent

Source: Adapted from Frances *et al.*, 1991.

defined spheres of authority, command-and-control leadership, an emphasis on rules, routines and standard operating procedures. Communication and co-ordination *between* agencies, as well as between functions and departments *within* bureaucracies were, however, problematic, leading to compartmentalised approaches to problems (departmental 'silos' and tunnel vision). In addition it was argued particularly by New Right commentators in the 1980s that large bureaucracies were inflexible in adapting to change, and their procedural emphasis bought at the expense of results.

In the 1980s and 1990s the perceived failings of bureaucracy led to a renewed emphasis on markets and competition in the delivery of public services. Conservative governments privatised large parts of the public sector, and exposed what was left to market disciplines through quasi-markets, compulsory competitive tendering, market testing and so on. Large multi-functional bureaucracies were broken up into a network of specialised agencies contracting for services with a variety of public, private and voluntary providers.

Under the market mode of governance co-ordination is achieved by the invisible hand of the market rather than the visible authority of management. Price mechanisms and contract law are the means for regulating relationships, with conflicts settled by haggling or recourse to the courts. In the ideal-type model, the potential of co-operative alliances between actors to produce synergies and/or increase market power is limited by suspicion of competitors and the preferences of actors for independent action and control. In reality, such alliances are increasingly common in the commercial world.

In the public sector, the introduction of competition proved to be a problematic exercise for many reasons (Ranade, 1998; Flynn *et al.*, 1996; Wistow *et al.*, 1996; Robinson and Le Grand, 1994) and always co-existed with strong hierarchical controls downwards from central government, notably in setting and regulating the performance targets expected from actors in the market. The break-up of bureaucracies introduced more actors into the policy arena, making co-ordination and a holistic approach to service delivery more difficult rather than less. Strategically this fragmentation also made the whole system more difficult to steer in any coherent direction. It was argued that competition and the 'contract culture' had promoted self-interested behaviour rather than the public interest, and low trust relationships rather than high trust.

By the late 1990s, and partly as a response to these issues, the emphasis changed to networks and partnerships as the dominant mode of co-ordination. However, the incoming Labour government did not return to the *status quo ante*. For example, it retained the purchaser and provider splits in health and social care and the approaches to contracting out in local authorities (without the compulsion), but exhorted and sometimes mandated agencies to collaborate to overcome the negative effects of fragmentation. (A statutory duty of partnership, for example, was laid on all health organisations.) There was also renewed emphasis on the role of the community and voluntary sectors as well as business as active policy partners with government. A plethora of new collaborative arrangements have since ensued in health, regeneration, economic development, social care, community safety and other fields.

The key feature of the network mode of governance is that co-ordination is achieved by less formal and more egalitarian means than the other two models, and explicit attention is paid to the way co-operation and trust are formed and maintained. Macneil (1985) has suggested that the 'entangling strings' of reputation, friendship, interdependence and altruism all become an integral part of the relationship, and that the information obtained is thereby both 'thicker' than that in the market and 'freer' than that communicated in a hierarchy. Where such a model can be created it has distinct advantages especially in relation to the exchange of commodities whose value cannot be easily produced or traded (such as 'know-how') or when dealing with issues where both solutions to problems and the behaviour needed to attain them are highly uncertain (Pratt et al., 1999). Rhodes (1997) argues that networks, as an increasingly important mode of social co-ordination in both public and private sectors, are also relatively autonomous and self-organising. The state can steer them by a variety of incentives and sanctions, but cannot totally control them.

Although useful up to a point, this chronological account, which superimposes changing modes of governance on different historical epochs, over-simplifies the real position. Rather than superseding each other as the dominant 'operating mode' of government, markets, hierarchy and networks have been *overlaid* on each other and *co-exist* in complex sets of relationships in different settings. Similar views have been expressed by others. For example, Martin (2000: 209) argues that we have now a hybrid model of governance which is characterised by 'the co-existence and interaction of hierarchical, market-based and collaborative frameworks' and Hoggett (1999: 24) argues that 'paradox and contradiction' govern the present restructuring of public services rather than the 'either-or binary logic of the past'.

At the same time, some writers have argued that modes of governance should not be confused with organisational form. In the real world organisations operate in 'mixed mode' (Bradach and Eccles, 1991) and, specifically, 'the multi-organisational partnership as an organisational form should not be confused with the network as a mode of governance' (Lowndes and Skelcher, 1998: 319). From their research on urban regeneration partnerships, Lowndes and Skelcher argue that different modes of governance characterise different stages in the lifecycle of partnerships. While the network mode with its emphasis on trust, informality and co-operation characterises the early and late stages of partnership formation and dissolution, hierarchy predominates as the partnership consolidates and formalises its operations, and the market mode with its associated behaviours dominates the stage of programme delivery, as providers compete for contracts and project grants.

This analysis gives the impression that actors choose from plural modes as appropriate in a rather sophisticated way, but to a large extent these are forced choices, resulting from the tensions and contradictions arising from the changes in public policy and management we have outlined. Modes of governance may not be the same as organisational form, but a particular mode is consistent with one form or another in terms of behaviour and operating assumptions. It is instructive, for instance, that in Lowndes and Skelcher's research 'many respondents saw networks as the life-blood of the partnership, pointing to the importance of sustaining these beneath the surface of increasingly bureaucratic and hierarchical arrangements' (Lowndes and Skelcher, 1998: 324). The increased scope and ambition of some of the new partnerships requires a very high level of collaborative commitment, as Pratt et al. (1999) point out, yet they too operate in the same hierarchical and marketised environment.

For example, in spite of New Labour's ambivalence about embracing the market in the delivery of public service, in practice they have been as supportive of the externalisation of local government services to private providers as their predecessors, through policies such as the Private Finance Initiative, Best Value and 'strategic service-providing partnerships' (Sillett, 2002; Whitehead, 2001; Grimshaw et al., 2002). Government policy has also propelled the voluntary sector into the mainstream of service delivery, in housing, social care, environmental services and community and economic regeneration programmes (Gastor and Deakin, 1998). The resulting fragmentation and contract culture works against the government's belief in a holistic approach to regeneration, service delivery and social inclusion. As Whitfield (2001) comments: 'this requires integrated teams, the pooling of skills, experience and resources between organisations in networks, partnerships, alliances and coalitions with the public sector playing a central role. It requires joined-up government, not joined-up contracts'.

Overlay this marketisation with the increasingly strong hierarchical approaches to performance management that this government has used with local government, the health service and executive agencies in recent years, and the contradictions facing multi-organisational partnerships are apparent, both in theory and practice. For example, how do organisations and individuals manage the tensions of being competitors for resources in one setting, and collaborators for the greater good in another? How are the flexibilities consistent with partnership working, affected by the strong hierarchical controls and performance targets laid on public organisations by national government? Can the inequalities of status and power which characterise relations in markets and bureaucracies be overcome in the more egalitarian ethos required of partnerships? And what incentives can persuade policy actors to give the voluntary commitment asked of them? Do notions of altruism and the 'public good' suffice? We explore some of these questions in more detail in the rest of the article.

FINDING A BASIS FOR COLLABORATION

As discussed earlier, organisational individualism is increasingly seen as an inadequate response to the growth in task scope (Alter and Hage, 1993) – that is, the degree to which a problem to be solved must be addressed from many perspectives. If greater knowledge persuades us to see problems as multi-faceted then we will be pushed into more complex kinds of collaborative mechanisms. Individualism is also seen as less appropriate in the public sector as opposed to the private sector. Indeed, the distinguishing feature of the public sector according to one influential account was its focus on inter-organisational linkages:

> good results depend on co-operation among many organisations with interdependent functions. ... It is intensive and sustained inter-organisational co-operation that is the hallmark of success in public management, rather than single-minded pursuit of individual organisational objectives. (Metcalfe and Richards, 1990: 237)

Having said that, the advantages of co-operation are increasingly heralded in the private sector as well and take a variety of forms as a response to the growth of global competition, speed of technological innovation and ease of technological transfer (Kantor, 1994). Companies are having to learn to 'manage through networks' (Lorenz, 1991; Snow et al., 1993) as their relationships with suppliers and distributors becomes more complex. This does not mean that competition ceases to be important. Instead strategies which decide on the basis of organisational self interest when an adversarial or co-operative stance is required is regarded by commentators as the optimal course of action for individual firms (what Burton (1995) calls a 'composite strategy'). Pratt et al. (1999) also argue that co-operation between firms is a way of dealing with an uncertain environment, and may arise entirely from considerations of self interest without any shared goals between the co-operators.[1]

But even if the climate is favourable, and collaboration is widely regarded as a virtue, finding a legitimate basis for collaboration may still be difficult. An important contribution to understanding why and in what circumstances collaboration is likely to occur is provided by Benson (1975) with his concept of *resource dependency*. Taking as his starting point the way in which organisations defend their own interests, and recognising the likelihood of conflict where such interests prove incompatible, he argues that:

> interactions at the level of service delivery are ultimately dependent upon resource acquisition. ... It is assumed that organisational decision-makers are typically oriented to the acquisition and defence of an adequate supply of resources. Two basic types of resources are central to the political economy of inter-organisational networks. These are money and authority. (p.231)

This basic organisational orientation leads to a number of decision criteria which govern inter-agency relations:

- *The fulfilment of programme requirements*: agencies are reluctant to undertake tasks or to tolerate practices which interfere with the fulfilment of present programmes.
- *The maintenance of a clear domain of high social importance*: agencies will seek to maintain uncluttered control over a key set of important activities. Such a domain is characterised by one or more of the following attributes – exclusiveness, autonomy and dominance.
- *The maintenance of orderly reliable patterns of resource flow*: organisations will endeavour to see that their support network operates in a predictable, dependable way permitting the agency to anticipate an adequate and certain flow of resources.
- *The extended application and defence of the agency's paradigm*: participants are committed to their agency's way of doing things, to its own definition of problems and tasks and its own techniques of intervention.

Benson also distinguishes between *equilibrium situations* where a policy domain is structured in such a way that the individual organisations are able to sustain adequate supplies of money and authority without competition or domain disputes, and *non-equilibrium situations* in which organisations are forced into competitive situations where they have to actively struggle to defend these resources. The implications of his analysis are that organisational life is marked by a constant struggle for survival and domain control, and collaboration will only be entered into where there is some mutual benefit to be derived from doing so.

The relevance of this analysis to our previous discussion is clear. The conscious introduction of markets and competition into the public sector in the 1980s and early 1990s, as well as threats to the exclusiveness and autonomy of *professional* domains (in medicine and teaching, for example) which also occurred and still continue, have disturbed the previous equilibrium, increasing competition for resources and the struggle to maintain domain control.

The possibilities for inter-agency collaboration to achieve collective goals for the public good appear to be limited in Benson's model, but can take place if there is a possibility of mutual gain. In particular Benson stresses that super-ordinate bodies can make a difference by structuring the local environment to provide a facilitating framework for collaboration. In addition, collaboration is more likely to occur if agencies are able to increase the efficiency with which scarce resources are used, or some additional resources are given, particularly when these are made conditional on the achievement of collaboration. It is precisely these kinds of incentives which have been made available in health and education action zones, and new regeneration and community-based initiatives. Nevertheless, while agencies may successfully collaborate to win such resources, it cannot be guaranteed that they will continue to work effectively to achieve their sometimes ambitious social or economic objectives over long time frames. As one of Lowndes and Skelchers' respondents put it: 'There's a vast difference between a package of money and real inter-agency working. You can have the first with outright enemies' (Lowndes and Skelcher, 1998: 327). Benson's analysis suggests that success is predicated, as in the private sector, on hard-headed deals which promise mutual gain.

OVERCOMING BARRIERS AND MANAGING CONTRADICTION

Even when there is a firm basis for collaboration, there are many barriers to overcome. Hardy *et al.* (1992) identify five categories of barrier as detailed in Figure 3. From the point of view of individual organisations, collaboration may pose a threat. Hudson (1987) identifies two main difficulties: each agency loses some of its freedom to act independently and must invest scarce resources in developing relationships with other organisations when the potential return on that investment is often unclear and intangible. It may also mean having to share the credit with other organisations for any achievements, or even letting another organisation take all the credit (Huxham and Macdonald, 1992). Charlesworth *et al.* (1996) refer here to the importance of distinctive organisational tensions between flexibility and control. The search for collaboration requires organisational flexibilities in the construction of joint agendas (thereby

FIGURE 3
FIVE CATEGORIES OF BARRIER TO COLLABORATION

Structural
Fragmentation of service responsibilities across inter-agency boundaries
Fragmentation of service responsibilities within agency boundaries
Inter-organisational complexity
Non-coterminosity of boundaries

Procedural
Differences in planning horizons and cycles
Differences in budgetory cycles and procedures

Financial
Differences in funding mechanisms and bases
Differences in the stocks and flows of resources

Professional
Differences in ideologies and values
Professional self-interest
Threats to job security
Conflicting views about user interests and roles

Status and Legitimacy
Organisational self interest
Concern for threats to autonomy and domain
Differences in legitimacy between elected and appointed agencies

Source: Hardy *et al.*, 1992.

surrendering a degree of definitional power), joint resourcing (surrendering a degree of resource control) and joint working (surrendering a degree of control over staff time, energy and corporate loyalty). To do so often requires a leap of faith and degree of trust not engendered by the 'contract culture'.

At the same time, organisations face stronger top-down imperatives to tighten control in the pursuit of their own strategic objectives and performance targets. If anything, these pressures have intensified since 1997. Hence public agencies face a two-way pressure – to deliver their core business targets and participate in inter-organisational partnerships. To the degree that partnership working is still seen as marginal to the 'real' business of the organisation in terms of rewards and resources, delivering on the core business will inevitably take precedence. Even when agencies do acknowledge the potential importance of a partnership in helping them deliver some of their own key objectives, in practice many experience frustration that the linkages do not happen. This quotation from a health authority manager in Ranade's research on a strategic health partnership illustrates these points:

The business that the Health Partnership wants to do isn't aligned properly with the business the health organisations want to do. Two meetings ago the main agenda item was domestic violence. Now whilst as a member of society and employee of the public sector I feel very strongly about domestic violence ... if I list the two hundred things I could get sacked for tomorrow, not doing something about domestic violence isn't one of them ... We can't commit and run to the fifty things the Partnership has brought up because the opportunity cost of not doing the other seventy-five means we won't have made as much progress with the national service framework on mental health or coronary heart disease or waiting lists and times.[2]

ISSUES OF MEMBERSHIP

The self-organising nature of networks means there are key questions over who is included and who is excluded. While governments can act to ensure the adequate representation of weaker stakeholders, and have done in many of the regeneration partnerships, this may still result in the development of relatively exclusive self-perpetuating groups forming, where the same people talk to each other in a variety of different locales. The emphasis on friendships, personal contact and informality in network-style relationships means that 'insider' and 'outsider' groups can form in partnerships. Poorly resourced or marginalised groups find it difficult to 'break in' to the networks, or get access to relevant, timely information, leading to suspicions that partnership decisions are 'sewn up' in advance between the insiders (Lowndes and Skelcher, 1998; Hastings, 1996).

The representation of voluntary and community groups on partnerships can be a particularly thorny issue, because of their size, diversity and varying mandates. Elected councillors and line-managed officers from public sector bureaucracies can be dismissive of the sources of their legitimacy or, by contrast, accord them a representativeness which they do not possess and feel uneasy about (the problem of the 'token' black, disabled or youth member). Ranade (2000) found that where the voluntary sector had effective mechanisms for aggregating and co-ordinating the views of its 'constituency of interest' its representatives could claim a more powerful mandate and authority in the strategic health partnership she studied, although individual personal characteristics were also important.

Some writers have argued that stakeholder analysis can be useful in helping convenors of partnerships identify who might have an interest in the partnership, or be able to affect it (Eden, 1996; Finn, 1996; Gray, 1996). This enables potential collaborators to be involved at appropriate stages, identifies potential supporters and saboteurs and suggests ways of managing stakeholders through the cultivation of alliances or other tactics.

DEVELOPING A COLLABORATIVE CULTURE

As discussed earlier, 'co-evolving' partnerships designed to tackle the 'wicked issues' presuppose a high level of collaborative commitment, and ways of working consistent with a network mode of governance. However, members bring with them into the collaboration the beliefs and behaviour which characterise their own organisation and relationships outside the partnership. For example:

- *Inequalities of status and power:* the underlying premise of co-evolving partnerships is that no one has a monopoly of knowledge about a problem and that everyone is part of the solution. Hence partnerships should work on the principle of the equal worth of each member's contribution. In practice, members import into partnerships the hierarchies of power, resources and status which exist outside, and the tensions and conflicts which mark these relationships. A key question concerns the extent to which 'those accustomed to being in control are willing to cede power to others' (Marsh and Beazeley, 1996: 4). Mackintosh (1992) argues that if gaining access to new resources is the prime goal of the partners, and 'added value' is perceived in strictly financial terms (resource synergies), the contribution of those not in control of large budgets will be devalued. 'Policy synergy', however, is more characteristic of co-evolving partnerships. Policy synergy concerns the involvement of partners in the policy process, with synergies derived from inherent differences or 'innovation due to complementary perspectives' (Hastings, 1996: 261) which tries to generate appropriate solutions to old problems. In this type of partnership the differences between the partners are reduced to some extent by mutual respect and empathy, and the desire to learn.

- *Styles of leadership:* co-evolving partnerships demand a different style of leadership from that associated with managing hierarchical organisations; facilitative rather than command and control (since membership is voluntary and organisations can walk away if they wish). Smith and Beazley (2002) argue that involvement is enhanced under conditions of 'policy synergy', and conditions are more inclusive and democratic. The concept of 'leadership' in these conditions is more diffuse and subtle (for example, see the discussion on reticulists and 'boundary spanners' below). People used to working in hierarchies may not have the requisite skills and qualities. The voluntary and community sector with their more egalitarian and participative ethos are a more likely source of facilitative leadership. Because they possess less resource and position power, they are forced to hone their skills of influence and persuasion. However, powerful senior executives from the statutory and private sectors, used to command and control in their own organisation, are unlikely to defer easily to others in a partnership, and struggles for leadership can seriously inhibit its development.

- *Scope and purpose:* most approaches to collaboration take it for granted that an explicit statement of shared purpose is a pre-requisite to success, although that might develop over time rather than at the outset (Mattesich and Monsey, 1992; Cropper, 1995; Hardy *et al.*, 1992). Clear goals and objectives help to clarify boundaries and commitments and provide a control against collaborative drift, but some commentators argue that a degree of ambiguity at the outset can help people buy in to the change process without necessarily addressing the conflicts of interest which change implies (Pettigrew *et al.*, 1992; Nocan, 1989). However, there is a danger in this that partnerships sign up to ambitious grand designs at an early stage, overestimating the collaborative capacity of the membership. This notion refers to the level of activity or degree of change a collaborative relationship is able to sustain without any partner losing a sense of security in the relationship. Demands can both under-reach or over-reach thresholds of capacity. An under-estimate means that collaborative effort is confined to marginal tasks; over-estimates lead to unrealistic assessments of what can be achieved within given timescales.

Building a collaborative culture and identity takes time and requires a realistic appraisal of the current state of commitment and readiness to change of partnership members. Newman (1994) identifies four dimensions which can be used to assess their capacity for collaboration. First, the way people identify their *roles*. The past decade has seen the erosion of many fixed identities based upon profession, function and role, and the collaborative imperative may represent a further challenge to such identities. Second, the *location of boundaries* within and between organisations. The public sector has already seen a weakening of previously fixed boundaries which should help to promote collaboration, but this depends on how staff at different levels adapt to this fluidity. Third, the way people construct *notions of progress* for themselves. The injunction to work collaboratively may represent a dynamic framework for progress and change for some, but others may see it as an attack on their specialisms and assumptions about the best interests of users. This relates to Newman's final dimension, a *sense of social purpose*, which has traditionally characterised many public sector organisations – people's sense of personal mission.

NURTURING AND RECOGNISING THE RETICULISTS

The discussion in managerialist literature of 'change champions' whose commitment and charisma become crucial to the successful development of collaborative initiatives, bears a strong relationship to the notion of 'reticulists' in the literature of policy analysis (Friend *et al.*, 1974). Reticulists are individuals with a strong commitment to change who act as 'entrepreneurs of power' (Degeling, 1995), skilled at mapping and developing policy networks, identifying where linkages and coupling are possible, able to build coalitions and alliances with other committed and powerful individuals in their own and other organisations.

Some but not all of these individuals have key roles to play managing across organisational boundaries as partnership co-ordinators or developers. 'Boundary spanners' (Ranade, 1998) will have rather different tasks from those with conventional line management functions within organisations. For example:

- Managing across and upwards, rather than downwards. Boundary spanners rarely manage large numbers of people.
- Influencing and motivating others over whom they have little control.
- Creating and assembling resources owned by others.
- Building trust between partners with different interests, perspectives and organisational imperatives.
- Achieving tangible outcomes, to keep members committed to the partnership while moving the wider agenda forward.
- Maintaining relationships and communication networks across agencies at a variety of levels.

The skills and characteristics of reticulists have not been widely researched,[3] although Ranade's small sample of boundary spanners all had long experience of inter-sectoral work, and possessed a wide range of inter-personal and social skills for what are essentially brokerage roles. These included:

- *Facilitation:* the boundary spanners often have highly developed skills as process experts and knowledge of the stages of partnership development. This knowledge also gave them greater patience about the time it takes for partnerships to start performing well.
- *Steering:* an ability to steer a group in more productive directions, by changing its focus or membership or linking it with more powerful or creative groups elsewhere in the system.
- *Negotiation:* political astuteness about the motivations and interests of other partners, combined with skills at negotiating 'win–win' agreements enabled them to keep a partnership moving forward even in difficult circumstances.

- *Communication and inter-personal skills:* an ability to relate easily to a wide variety of people at different levels and communicate clearly and in a manner appropriate to the audience was clearly important.
- *Entrepreneurship:* creating and assembling resources to make progress on innovative projects or fledgling initiatives.
- *Mediation*: boundary spanners can play an important role in explaining and interpreting a partner's behaviour and resolving conflicts and misunderstandings.

Perhaps the most noteworthy feature of all the respondents was their ability to combine a broad strategic vision of what their partnership should be trying to achieve, with flexible and pragmatic tactics in dynamic situations.

By the nature of their commitment to collaboration, boundary spanners appear to develop more complex models of social problems, and broader, more inclusive solutions than the more restricted perspectives of any one profession or agency. If this involves giving up turf and territory faster than others in their organisation can tolerate, there are dangers of being disowned and punished. The dangers are greatest for individuals trying to bridge the gap between statutory agencies and disadvantaged groups who may be deeply distrustful of officialdom. Maintaining the balance between being a constructive partner, yet not being co-opted, and maintaining the trust of local groups is difficult (for an illustration, see Stewart and Ranade, 2001).

In their analysis of network organisations in the private sector, Snow *et al.* (1993) identify very similar roles to the reticulists, with similar skills and abilities. However, they break it down into more specialised components, identifying three types of 'broker' role which are crucial to the success of the network, relating to network design, network operations and network maintenance. The first two overlap and may be undertaken by the same person and the authors identify entrepreneurial, negotiating and contractual skills as key requirements. The third, the network caretaker, has the function of maintaining and enhancing the network, developing a sense of community among its members. 'Networks operate effectively when member firms voluntarily behave as if they are all part of a broader organisation sharing common objectives and rewards' (Snow *et al.*, 1993: 34). The authors claim it is the most challenging role but the least understood, and it is by no means easy to say what kind of background such individuals will come from, or the training they require. The boundary spanners in Ranade's research were located in health, local government and the voluntary and community sectors. Those from statutory organisations complained that the time taken to perform the 'network caretaking' role was never acknowledged or supported by their bosses. Paradoxically, the value of this work was only acknowledged when illness or maternity leave disrupted it, and in one case led to a near-breakdown of communications between two organisations.

What does seem clear is that reticulists must begin from a sound position of power and legitimacy. McCann and Gray (1986) use the term 'convenor legitimacy' and identify several aspects of this status: a perception by others as having sufficient legitimacy to assume the role; being perceived as unbiased and able to manage multiple points of view; a vision or sense about the critical issues and first steps which need to be taken; previous experience of an inter-agency approach; participatory development style; and political skills which encourage others to take risks. It is, however, far from evident that these qualities are readily available or equally distributed within and between agencies. It is also evident that where collaborative initiatives do arise from reticulist activity, they need to be protected against the possibility of the departure of the key actors (Hardy et al., 1996). The link between the unplanned movement of key personnel and the draining of energy, purpose, commitment and action from major change processes has been established from a range of studies (Goodman and Dean, 1982; Kanter, 1985; Pettigrew, 1985).

TRANSACTION COSTS OF NETWORKS AND PARTNERSHIPS

A key criticism in the literature on quasi-markets in health and social care related to the transaction costs involved in the specification, negotiation and monitoring of contracts (see, e.g., Le Grand and Bartlett, 1991). Yet the transaction costs of partnerships and networks may be equally high. Huxham (1996) argues that the danger of 'collaborative inertia' is ever present. The time and effort required to agree even trivial things, create more understanding about each partner's perspective or negotiate a common purpose can break the will of even the most committed collaborator. Multiply this effort by the number of new partnership initiatives which have been spawned in the last few years and the transaction costs of the collaborative imperative appear to require more serious study and assessment.

The costs of partnership working also bear heavily on those least able to bear them. Voluntary sector agencies may have insufficient administrative capacity to engage effectively with partnerships and carry out their core work (Lowndes et al., 1997; Ranade, 2000) and community representatives may be giving their time unpaid.

CONCLUSION

The rhetoric which currently surrounds inter-organisational collaboration as an attractive ideal cloaks the fact that the network mode of social organisation coexists with, and is embedded in, other modes based on hierarchies and markets. A conceptual exploration which starts from this premise can provide a more realistic analysis of some of the factors which inhibit partnership development, and better understanding by the participants of the issues real partnerships need to address if they are to achieve their collaborative potential.

To argue that a network mode of governance is well suited to addressing the 'wicked issues' is not to suggest that hierarchy and markets have no role to play. Since so much of the empirical literature on networks has stemmed from studies of firms and businesses, the emphasis had tended to be on the factors that produce, develop and sustain *voluntary* relationships. However, much of the public policy agenda has been *mandated* to varying degrees by a central executive authority – central government – and *imposed* upon local agencies. The question is not so much whether hierarchies, markets and networks can co-exist, (because clearly they do), but rather the extent to which they can do so effectively. Networks cannot be created by administrative fiat, but hierarchy can create a context in which such developments might be more likely to arise. If New Labour acknowledges this as the limit of its hierarchical remit, and then encourages and facilitates a network approach in localities, removing some of the more obvious hurdles and contradictions emanating from their own actions, there is some chance of further progress. If it sticks to the idea that it can control the whole 'partnership show' by centrally determined incentives, targets and policy approaches it will achieve little more than a cosmetic gain. Equally, enthusiasts of a network approach cannot reasonably expect to be left alone to develop voluntary, self-directed exchanges as and when they think fit. The most productive route is likely to be a 'loose–tight' configuration offering localities a great deal of freedom to do their own thing, but always within a framework of mutually agreed values and standards. As Rhodes (1997) has argued, 'it's the mix that matters'.

NOTES

1. A considerable body of literature has arisen on the conditions which promote such co-operation. Probably the most influential is Axelrod's *The Evolution of Co-operation* (1990), which describes the game of the iterated Prisoner's Dilemma.
2. Unpublished quotation from research interview, Ranade, 2000.
3. Further recent research on 'boundary spanners' is reported in Williams (2002). The skills and competencies identified by the author parallel very closely those discussed here.

REFERENCES

Alter, C. and J. Hage, 1993, *Organisations Working Together* (California: Sage).

Axelrod, R., 1990, *The Evolution of Co-operation* (London: Penguin).

Benson, J.K., 1975, 'The Inter-Organisational Network as a Political Economy', *Administrative Science Quarterly*, 20 (June), pp.229–49.

Booth, T., 1988, *Developing Policy Research* (Aldershot: Gower).

Bradach, J. and R. Eccles, 1991, 'Price, Authority and Trust: From Ideal Types to Plural Forms', in G. Thompson, J. Frances, R. Levacic and J. Mitchell (eds.), *Markets, Hierarchies and Networks, the Co-ordination of Social Life* (London: Sage).

Burton, J., 1995, 'Composite Strategy: The Combination of Collaboration and Competition', *Journal of General Management*, 21/1, pp.1–23.

Capra, F., 1997, *The Web of Life* (London: Harper Collins).

Challis, L. *et al.*, 1988, *Joint Approaches to Social Policy: Rationality and Practice* (Cambridge: Cambridge University Press).

Charlesworth, J., J. Clarke and A. Cochrane, 1996, 'Tangled Webs? Managing Local Mixed Economies of Care', *Public Administration*, 74 (Spring), pp.67–88.

Cropper, S., 1995, 'Collaborative Working and the Issue of Sustainability', in Huxham, 1995.

Degeling, P., 1995, 'The Significance of "Sectors" in Calls for Urban Public Health Inter-Sectoralism: An Australian Perspective', *Policy and Politics*, 23/4, pp.289–301.

Department of Environment, Transport and the Regions, 1998, *Modernising Local Government: Local Democracy and Community Leadership* (London: HMSO).

Eden, C, 1995, 'The Stakeholder/Collaborator Workshop', in Huxham, 1995.

Finn, C.B., 1995, 'Utilising Stakeholder Strategies for Positive Collaborative Outcomes', in Huxham 1995.

Flynn, R., G. Williams and S. Pickard, 1996, *Markets and Networks: Contracting in Community Health Services* (Buckingham: Open University Press).

Frances, J., R. Levacic, J. Mitchell and G. Thompson, 1991, 'Introduction', in G. Thompson, J. Frances, R. Levacic and J. Mitchell (eds.), *Markets, Hierarchies and Networks: The Coordination of Social Life* (London: Sage).

Friend, J., J. Power and C. Yewlett, 1974, *Public Planning: The Inter-Corporate Dimension* (London: Tavistock).

Goodman, P.S. and J.W. Dean, 1982, 'Creating Long-Term Organisational Change', in P.S. Goodman (ed.), *Change in Organisations* (San Francisco: Jossey Bass).

Gray, B., 1995, 'Cross-Sectoral Partners: Collaborative Alliances among Business, Government and Communities' in Huxham, 1995.

Grimshaw, D., S. Vincent and H. Willmott, 2002, 'Going Privately: Partnership and Outsourcing in UK Public Services', *Public Administration*, 80/3, pp.475–502.

Hardy, B., A. Turrell and G. Wistow, 1992, *Innovations in Community Care Management* (Aldershot: Avebury).

Hastings, A., 1996, 'Unravelling the Process of "Partnership" in Urban Regeneration Policy', *Urban Studies*, 33/2, pp.253–68.

Hoggett, P., 1996, 'New Modes of Control in the Public Sector', *Public Administration*, 74, pp.9–32.

Hudson, B., 1987, 'Collaboration in Social Welfare: A Framework for Analysis', *Policy and Politics*, 15/3, pp.175–8.

Hudson, B., 1999, 'Primary Health Care and Social Care: Working across Professional Boundaries', *Managing Community Care*, 7/1, pp.15–22.

Hudson, B., R. Young, B. Hardy and C. Glendinning, 2001, *National Evaluation of Notifications for Use of the Section 31 Partnership Flexibilities of the Health Act 1999, Second Interim Report* (Leeds and Manchester: Nuffield Institute for Health/National Primary Care Research and Development Centre).

Huxham, C. (ed), 1995, *Creating Collaborative Advantage* (Sage: London).

Huxham, C. and D. Macdonald, 1992, 'Introducing Collaborative Advantage', *Management Decision*, 30/3, pp.50–56.

Kanter, R.M., 1984, *The Change Masters* (London: Unwin).

50   PARTNERSHIPS BETWEEN HEALTH AND LOCAL GOVERNMENT

Lorenz, E., 1991, 'Neither Friends nor Strangers: Informal Networks of Subcontracting in French Industry', in G. Thompson *et al.* (eds.), *Markets, Hierarchies and Networks* (London: Sage).
Lowndes, V., A. McCabe and C. Skelcher, 1996, 'Networks, Partnership and Urban Regeneration', *Local Economy*, 11/4, pp.333–42.
Lowndes, V. and C. Skelcher, 1998, 'The Dynamics of Multi-Organisational Partnerships: An Analysis of Changing Modes of Governance', *Public Administration*, 76 (Summer), pp.313–33.
Mackintosh, M., 1992, 'Partnership: Issues of Policy and Negotiation', *Local Economy*, 7/3, pp.210–24.
Macneil, I., 1985, 'Relational Contract', *Wisconsin Law Review*, 3, pp.483–526.
Marsh, A. and M. Beazeley, 1996, 'Urban Regeneration and the Community', Paper presented to the School of Public Policy Conference on the Changing Nature of Public Management, University of Birmingham, 24–25 Jan.
Martin, S., 2000, 'Implementing "Best Value": Local Public Services in Transition', *Public Administration*, 78/1, pp.209–27.
McCann, J. and B. Gray, 1986, 'Power and Collaboration in Human Service Domains', *International Journal of Sociology and Social Policy*, 6, pp.58–67.
Montesich, P. and B. Monsey, 1992, *Collaboration: What Makes It Work?* (St. Paul, MN: Alder H. Wilder Foundation).
Pettigrew, A., 1985, *The Awakening Giant: Continuity and Change in ICI* (Oxford: Basil Blackwell).
Pettigrew, A., E. Ferlie and L. McKee, 1992, *Shaping Strategic Change* (London: Sage).
Pratt, J., D. Plamping and P. Gordon, 1998, *Partnership: Fit for Purpose?* (London: King's Fund).
Pratt, J., D. Plamping and P. Gordon, 1999, *Working Whole Systems: Putting Theory into Practice in Organisations* (London: King's Fund).
Metcalfe, L., and S. Richard, 1990, *Improving Public Management* (European Institute of Public Administration, Sage).
Newman, J., 1994, 'Beyond the Vision: Cultural Change in the Public Sector', *Public Money and Management* (April/June), pp.59–64.
Nocan, A, 1989, 'Forms of Ignorance and their Role in the Joint Planning Process', *Social Policy and Administration*, 23/1, pp.31–47.
Ranade, W., 2000, *Developing the Voluntary Sector in Health*. Report to Newcastle Health Partnership
Ranade, W., 1998, *Making Sense of Multi-Agency Groups* (Newcastle: Sustainable Cities Research Institute, University of Northumbria).
Ranade, W., 1998, 'Reforming the British National Health Service: All Change, No Change?' in Ranade, W. (ed), *Markets and Health Care: A Comparative Analysis* (London: Addison Wesley Longman).
Rhodes, R.A.W., 1997, *Understanding Governance* (Buckingham: Open University Press).
Rhodes, R.A.W., 1997b, 'From Marketisation to Diplomacy: It's the Mix that Matters', *Public Policy and Administration*, 12/2, pp.31–50.
Robinson, R. and J. Le Grand, 1994, *Evaluating the NHS Reforms* (London: King's Fund).
Sillett, J., 2001, *Public Private Partnership: Opening the Public Private Debate* (London: Local Government Information Unit).
Smith, M. and M. Beazley, 2000, 'Progressive Regimes, Partnerships and the Involvement of Local Communities: A Framework for Evaluation', *Public Administration*, 78/4 (Winter), pp.879–96.
Snow, C.C., R. Miles and H. Coleman, 1993, 'Managing 21st Century Network Organisations', in C. Mabey and B. Mayon-White (eds.), *Managing Change* (London: Paul Chapman Press).
Stewart, B. and W. Ranade, 2001, 'Taking the Heat: Resolving Conflict Through a Partnership Approach', *Local Governance*, 27/4, pp.213–21.
Whitehead, A., 2001, 'Clearing up the Dogma Doings – Labour and the Market', *Renewal*.
Whitfield, D., 2001, *Public Services and Corporate Welfare* (Pluto Press).
Wistow, G. *et al.*, 1996, *Social Care Markets: Problems and Prospects* (Buckingham).
Williams, P., 2002, 'The Competent Boundary Spanner', *Public Administration*, 80/1, pp.103–25.

Joint Working:
The Health Service Agenda

CAROLINE GLENDINNING
and ANNA COLEMAN

CAROLINE GLENDINNING
and ANNA COLEMAN

SETTING THE SCENE – NEW LABOUR AND THE NHS

From GP Fund-Holding to Primary Care Groups and Trusts
Both the National Health Service (NHS) and its inter-organisational
relationships are major arenas for political activity and associated policy-
making by the Labour government. Within seven months of coming to
power in May 1997 a White Paper was published which proposed major
structural changes within the NHS in England (Secretary of State for
Health, 1997). These changes aimed to implement the Labour party's
election promise to end the politically divisive and allegedly inequitable
system of GP fund-holding and to 'renew the NHS as a genuinely national
service' (Ham, 1999: 55). The 1997 White Paper therefore announced the
end of GP fund-holding, but nevertheless retained the split between
purchasers and providers of health services. Indeed, it extended and
universalised the principle which had underpinned GP fund-holding –
devolving decisions about resource investment and service developments to
front-line primary health service professionals – to *all* family doctors and
community health services, through the creation of Primary Care Groups
(and subsequently Primary Care Trusts):

> In paving the way for the new NHS the Government is committed to
> building on what has worked but discarding what has failed ... Instead
> there will be a 'Third Way' of running the NHS – a system based on
> partnership and driven by performance ... It will be neither the model
> from the late 1970s nor the model from the early 1990s ... This Third
> Way builds on the successes that commissioning groups and
> fundholders have achieved over recent years. (Secretary of State for
> Health, 1997:10–27 passim)

Part of the reasoning behind this pragmatism, it has been argued, was to
avoid conflict with the medical profession, particularly those articulate,
'leading edge' general practitioners (GPs) who had enthusiastically
embraced fund-holding.

The New NHS Organisational Structures – Primary Care Groups and Trusts

Primary Care Groups and Trusts (PCG/Ts) bring together all the providers of primary and community health services (GPs, practice-based services, community nurses and other community health services) within a locality. PCGs were governed by boards, formally constituted as sub-committees of the local health authority and dominated by health and other professional (particularly GP) interests. Following their creation in April 1999, PCGs were expected to develop organisational capacity, expertise and growing autonomy, eventually becoming free-standing NHS Primary Care Trusts (PCTs). In an accelerated process of organisational development, all PCGs became Trusts in April 2002, when health authorities were abolished. The former PCG boards became the professional executive committees of PCTs, responsible for the day-to-day management of the organisation. PCTs have an additional, overarching board, similar to other NHS trusts, and are accountable for their performance to the new Strategic Health Authorities. PCTs (and PCGs before them) have three core responsibilities:

- Improving the health of the local population and reducing health inequalities.
- Developing primary and community health services.
- Commissioning community and hospital services.

PCG/Ts[1] are responsible for a single, unified budget covering hospital and community health services, prescribing and general practice infrastructure; together this accounts for about three-quarters of the total NHS budget for England. The unified budget is intended to create greater flexibility and improve opportunities for making major strategic shifts in service investment and expenditure (Paton, 1999). The aim of involving front-line health professionals, the size and scope of PCG/Ts' responsibilities, and their new accountability arrangements all have important implications for the ways in which NHS organisations and staff approach the collaborative agenda and for the potential success of these collaborations.[2]

In creating Primary Care Groups (PCGs), the government aimed to 'build on the experience of previous initiatives that had involved primary care professionals in the process of shaping and negotiating local patterns of service provision' (Goodwin, 2001: 4). Behind this lies a broader aim, which predates the current government, of pushing 'decision making down to the front-line worker, here the doctor, who is conceived to be closer to the needs and wishes of the consumer' (Walby and Greenwell, 1994: 60). However, this devolution also has the consequence of constraining the freedoms of professionals, through engaging them directly in the management of budgetary and normative constraints and ensuring compliance by their peers:

> professional autonomy has been a necessary casualty in a rationalising movement which has tried to manage resources with greater efficiency, establish a more pluralistic determination of priorities and more recently regulate standards of professional performance more effectively. (North and Peckham, 2001: 430; see also Croxon *et al.*, 2003)

From Treating to Preventing Illness

The Labour government made a distinctive break with past policies in its acknowledgement of widening inequalities in health, morbidity and mortality, and its recognition of the contributions of social, economic and environmental factors in these inequalities. These links were endorsed in a Green Paper on public health (DH, 1999a) and the subsequent White Paper *Saving Lives: Our Healthier Nation* (Secretary of State for Health, 1999). In order to tackle these inequalities, action at individual and community levels was advocated (broader, national and global activities to combat widening inequalities of wealth and income were eschewed) (Paton, 1999) and new responsibilities were assigned to local NHS organisations, in partnership with local authority, voluntary and community sector organisations. From 1999, PCG/Ts were required to develop explicit proposals for reducing health inequalities through their Health Improvement Plans (HImPs), to which local authorities were also signatories. In 2001, HImPs were renamed Health Improvement and Modernisation Plans (HIMPs), signifying an attempt to align local activities to tackle health improvement and health inequalities more closely with other organisational changes within the NHS; however, they remain the main vehicle for strategic planning by local NHS organisations and their partner organisations, particularly local authorities. According to the Department of Health (2001a), HIMPs should underpin and reflect the strategic plans of the Local Strategic Partnership (LSP) in the area to ensure that local health systems become key stake holders in LSPs.

The term 'health improvement' has numerous shades of meaning which are reflected both in official policy documents and in its usage by local organisations and professionals (Abbott and Gillam, 2000; Peckham, 2003). Nevertheless, its emergence signifies a distinctive new role for NHS organisations and professionals, whose responsibilities now include preventing ill-health as well as treating ill-health after it has arisen. Extensive inter-sectoral collaboration by NHS organisations is strongly advocated as the means for executing these new responsibilities.

The Drive for Implementation

The 1997 NHS White Paper was succeeded by a stream of further policy documents and prescriptions. In summer 2000, impatient with the pace of change, the government initiated a further strategic policy 'push', with the publication of the NHS Plan for England, containing targets and new implementation timetables in key health service areas such as intermediate care, access to hospital services, the quality of hospital care and preventable morbidity. In pursuit of these new targets, the NHS Plan promised substantial new funding (NHS, 2000), combined with the strengthening of regulatory and performance management mechanisms (Iliffe, 2001). In particular, very considerable emphasis was placed on collaboration between health and local authority services in order to prevent avoidable hospital admissions; expedite the discharge from hospital of older people whose medical treatment is complete; and invest in 'intermediate' rehabilitation and convalescence services. These goals were further reinforced by the publication in 2001 of a National Service Framework for Older People (DH, 2001b). Together, these processes and objectives are increasingly referred to as 'modernising' the NHS – the updating of services to increase their efficiency and responsiveness to users.

However, throughout the period, considerable tension has been apparent between the rhetoric of devolved local freedoms and professional empowerment; and the role of central government setting national policy agendas and targets to ensure the creation of uniformly high quality and equitable services across the country as a whole (see Dowling and Glendinning, 2003). This tension and its impact on NHS approaches to collaboration will be discussed in more detail below.

From Competition to Compulsory Collaboration

During its first term, the Labour government's aims for the NHS were intrinsically bound up with a new agenda for collaboration and 'partnership' working, in contrast to the allegedly 'adversarial' and certainly fragmented nature of the previous, market-driven NHS. However, these exhortations to collaboration extended much wider than just NHS and local government organisations. They reflect an overarching preoccupation with policy co-ordination and 'joined up government', from the Cabinet and Whitehall to co-ordinated initiatives and activities involving a wide range of statutory, voluntary and private organisations at local levels (Newman, 2001). One example is LSPs, which are intended to be cross-agency umbrella partnerships that include all sectors (private, public, community and voluntary) with a remit to work together to improve the life of a particular locality (DETR, 2001).

Nevertheless, the pressures on NHS and local authorities to engage in collaborative working have been particularly intense, prompting Paton (1999: 69) to refer to the 'oxymoron of "statutory voluntarism" ... in which partnership, co-operation and collaboration are emphasised and mandated at every turn'. Thus, since their creation PCG/Ts have been under a statutory duty to work in partnership; PCG boards and now the professional executive committees of PCTs are required to include a representative from the local social services department; and funding has been allocated in successive budgets and comprehensive spending reviews for local authority social services departments to develop joint activities with health partners.

At a strategic level, partnerships between NHS and local authorities have been underpinned by the latter's contribution to the development and implementation of local Health Improvement Plans (HImPs) and Health Improvement and Modernisation Plans (HIMPs); by the requirement for both sectors to collaborate together in local leadership of national service priorities (DH, 1998); and in preparing Joint Investment Plans for services for older people and other groups of users (DH, 2000).

The 1999 Health Act removed a number of structural barriers that were widely believed to impede both strategic and operational-level collaboration. The 'flexibilities' introduced by the Health Act allow NHS and local authorities to pool budgets for specific services (with the added freedom that the services purchased from a pooled budget do not need to reflect the proportional contributions of health and local authority organisations to that budget); to delegate statutory responsibility for commissioning services to one 'lead' organisation; and/or to integrate health and social services within a single organisational and managerial structure. Although the flexibilities extend across all local authority services, social services departments are virtually the only local authority services involved; in only one or two sites are other services such as housing, education or leisure also involved in these new integrated arrangements (Glendinning et al., 2002).

Health scrutiny is a further mechanism that extends local authority involvement in the NHS. Overview and scrutiny committees within social services local authorities have, since January 2003, a remit to scrutinise local health services as well as those for which the local authority is responsible. This gives added power to local authorities' responsibilities for promoting well-being and activity and is likely to include looking at health inequalities and health promotion as well as the planning, commissioning and provision of services. Health scrutiny provides an opportunity to take a cross-cutting view of local health needs and services. Guidance (DH, 2002) describes the purpose of health scrutiny as: 'Acting as a lever to improve the health of local people ... and securing the continuous improvement of health services and services that impact on health.'

Since the turn of the new century, the government has taken further the active promotion of partnerships between NHS and local authorities and 'spelled out a much harsher message for health service workers than that underpinning the earlier "partnership" model, calling for a new realism on the part of health professionals' (Newman, 2001: 92). The 2000 NHS Plan asserted the need for still closer operational links between health and social services staff; proposed a new cluster of financial incentives and rewards for joint working; and announced a new statutory partnership body, the Care Trust, whose governance arrangements reflect equal health and social services involvement and which can commission and provide integrated health and social services for specific groups of patients (DH, 2001c). Where collaboration is judged inadequate or ineffective, powers in the Health and Social Care Act 2001 allow the Secretary of State to require reluctant local partners to use the 1999 Health Act flexibilities (NHS, 2000). A further strong push for NHS and local authority services to collaborate over the improvement of hospital discharge arrangements and intermediate care services has been created by the intention in 2004 to impose charges on local authorities for delays in discharging people from hospital (Secretary of State, 2002). Yet further central government resources have been allocated to local authorities to enable them to build up convalescence and other support services and to develop smooth patient pathways in advance of this measure. Together, these measures pave the way for the increasing integration – whether voluntary or imposed – of health and local authority services, from linkage, through co-ordination, to full integration at the top of the collaborative ladder (Leutz, 1999).

The fervour with which current policies encourage collaboration between NHS and local authority organisations reflects the mutual interdependence of the two sectors and in particular the potential impact of this interdependence on some very high profile policy and political goals. For example, the 'modernisation' of the NHS includes demonstrating improved performance and greater efficiency in the use of acute hospital resources, as measured, for example, in reduced waiting lists and other waiting times for treatment. In turn, this involves preventing the hospital admission of people who could be treated or supported in other ways and discharging quickly those who no longer need acute medical care. However, achieving this level of efficiency depends on the availability of local authority funding and services to support frail and disabled people outside acute hospital settings; and collaboration with wider local authority and voluntary sector initiatives to maximise independence and prevent ill-health in the first place. The interdependencies between health and social services therefore have exceptionally high political salience. This makes them a key focus for 'political hyperactivism' – when 'politicians individually and collectively gain "points" with the media and party colleagues from making new initiatives almost for their own sake' (Dunleavy, 1995: 61). These inextricable linkages between politics and policies confound attempts at evaluation, particularly evaluations of the effectiveness or otherwise of particular policy initiatives. It becomes difficult to disentangle the impacts of different policy interventions and attribute changes to the impact of one, rather than any other initiative (or, indeed, combinations of measures). An additional risk is the marginalisation of longer term, developmental, strategies to improve health and well-being, in order to demonstrate improvements in shorter term (and more easily measurable) service productivities.

Two key issues can be identified which, it is argued, are likely to have a major impact on the range of collaborative activities between local authorities and NHS organisations: the changing organisational structures within the NHS and the extent to which primary care professionals are actively involved in the governance of PCG/Ts; and managerial pressures to deliver rapid evidence of 'modernisation' through improved performance, collaborative or otherwise.

RESEARCH EVIDENCE

Evidence on the progress of these developments is drawn from a longitudinal survey of a nationally representative sample of 15 per cent of English PCG/Ts. Postal, telephone and face-to-face interviews were carried out with key stake-holders (chairs, chief executives and other Board members) in autumn 1999 (Wilkin *et al.*, 2000), autumn 2000 (Wilkin *et al.*, 2001) and spring 2002 (Wilkin *et al.*, 2002). Other evidence comes from an evaluation of localities using the new Health Act flexibilities to integrate services (Glendinning *et al.*, 2002); and from the first stages of a study of health scrutiny (Coleman and Glendinning, forthcoming).

The Size, Structure and Responsibilities of PCG/Ts

The size of PCG/Ts and the scale of their activities offer new opportunities for overcoming the fragmentation inherent in general practice-based primary care. PCTs cover all GPs within a locality – membership is not optional – and are responsible for commissioning and providing services for an average of 150,000 patients (Wilkin *et al.*, 2002). Collaboration between neighbouring PCG/Ts, particularly over activities such as commissioning specialist services, increases yet further the size of the populations for which they may be responsible.

It is not simply their size that is significant, but the fact that PCG/Ts are corporate organisations with their own management and administrative staff; large, devolved, unified budgets; and explicit responsibilities for the health of, and services for, a whole area, rather than (as with general practice) small groups of registered patients. The number of staff employed by each PCT reflects the size of the population covered by the organisation and their extensive responsibilities and obligations; by 2002 the average number of management, financial and administrative staff employed by PCTs was 31.5 (Wilkin *et al.*, 2002).

The unified budgets held by PCTs, determined through a combination of weighted capitation and historic spending patterns, are substantial. Budgets are made up of elements which could previously only be spent in the separate areas of hospital and community health services; prescribed medication; and 'cash-limited GMS' (general medical services) funds, used to support GP practice infrastructure (premises, equipment and support staff). These unified budgets are free from the restrictions which previously constrained their expenditure: 'within this single cash envelope PCGs will be able to deploy the resources to best meet the health needs of their population' (HSC, 1998: 3).

PCTs' unified budgets offer unprecedented opportunities for making strategic shifts between different areas of health services expenditure. By 2002, some PCG/Ts had already made changes in the pattern of spending between different budget heads and most were planning such changes in the future. The main trend was towards increased spending on primary and community health services, often funded by reduced expenditure on hospital provision. Although this shift happens to reflect the interests of GPs, there is nevertheless evidence that PCTs are beginning to think strategically about their management of the unified budget (Dowling *et al.*, 2003). Other commentators suggest that the flexibility offered by PCG/Ts' devolved, integrated funding streams will lead to greater integration between primary, community and secondary health services (Goodwin, 2001).

PCG/Ts' governance and management structures are at least as important as their overall size. There are now several instances of a single chief executive being appointed to run both a PCT and a coterminous local authority or social service department (*The Guardian*, 14 May 2003) and numerous instances of joint appointments or secondments between PCTs and their social services or wider local authority partners.

The population-level responsibilities of PCG/Ts are reflected in their approaches to assessing the health needs of local people and commissioning services to meet those needs – in contrast to GP fund-holding, which 'was by definition atomized and responded mainly to the needs of individual patients' (North and Peckham, 2001: 430). By autumn 2001 a majority of PCG/Ts had carried out systematic assessments of local health needs,

FIGURE 1
HEALTH NEEDS ASSESSMENTS CARRIED OUT BY PCG/Ts (1999/2000/2002)

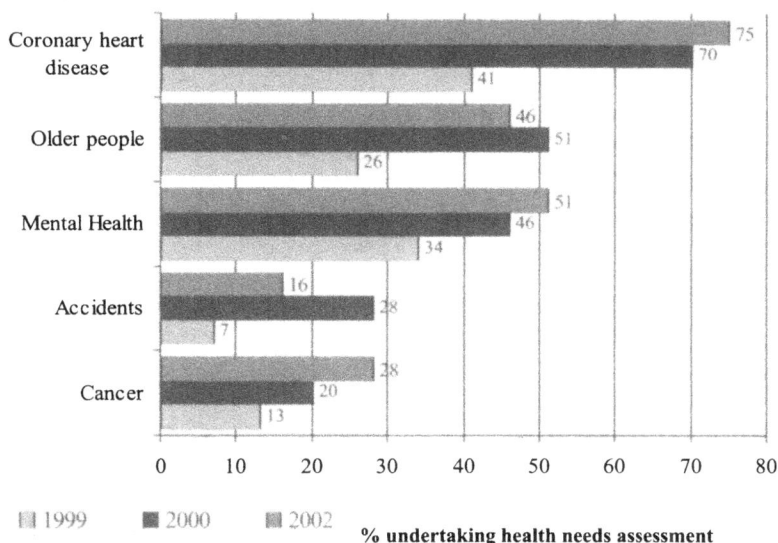

■ 1999   ■ 2000   ▨ 2002

% undertaking health needs assessment

especially in the priority areas of coronary heart disease, mental health and older people's services (Figure 1). This population perspective is likely to acquire even greater prominence following the abolition of health authorities in 2002 and the devolution to PCTs of all public health responsibilities – although there is little evidence from previous research or practice that either primary care organisations or professionals have the capacity or the inclination to do this (Peckham, 2003).

PCTs are also responsible for implementing a new system of clinical governance – a systematic approach to developing and monitoring the clinical and service standards of their professional providers. Clinical governance presents major challenges to the traditional professional autonomy of GPs (and to a lesser extent community-based nurses) and their claims to self-regulation (North and Peckham, 2001). Within their first 18 months, PCG/Ts had established systems for clinical governance; involved a wide range of staff and GP practices in clinical governance activities; and initiated educational approaches to improving quality of services. By 2002, 65 per cent of PCG/Ts were using financial incentive mechanisms to implement clinical governance (Wilkin *et al.*, 2002; Campbell and Roland, 2003). Although it remains to be demonstrated that these initiatives actually improve service quality, they will undoubtedly contribute to major cultural change, particularly among doctors and nurses in primary care, and a greater emphasis on managers and the public, as opposed to peer professional, accountability.

PCG/Ts and Partnerships with Local Authorities: Context and Challenges

Given their organisational form, size and responsibilities, the creation of PCG/Ts has also provided an unprecedented new opportunity to develop collaborative activities with local authority counterparts. Numerous earlier attempts to break down the 'Berlin Wall' between health and social services met with only limited success. Joint care planning teams and joint consultative committees were established in the late 1970s to facilitate the transfer of patients and resources from long-stay learning disability and mental illness hospitals to the community. However, although these structures were mandatory, it was not always easy for partners to agree on the aims or desirable outcomes of the collaboration. Differences in organisational structures, planning cycles, methods of allocating and auditing budgets and geographical boundaries all created additional barriers (Audit Commission, 1986). Consequently, although joint planning was often successful in relation to specific, small-scale and marginal activities, its impact on the strategic functions and mainstream activities of both health and social organisations was negligible (Nocon, 1994).

Most significantly, GPs, community nursing services, housing departments and other local authority services – all of which are, arguably, crucial to the provision of comprehensive non-institutional care – were marginal or absent from many of the initiatives of the 1980s and 1990s aiming to improve collaboration and service integration. Thus, local authority social services departments were simply obliged to 'consult' with health authorities and family health services authorities in preparing their community care plans; they were not required to involve them as partners. Care management, mandated upon local authority social services departments by the 1990 NHS and Community Care Act, was intended to enable individually tailored 'packages' of services to be purchased to meet the needs of individual users. However, in practice, care managers had no access to resources or services which were funded or provided by the NHS: 'SSDs had no power to require the involvement of any other agency or profession in the process. In the absence of a single health and social care budget, individual care managers were no more able to commit resources for a unified package of care than their predecessors' (Hudson, 1999: 191).

GPs complained about the lack of effective communication over the new community care arrangements (North and Peckham, 2001). Conversely, social services managers and professionals lamented the difficulty of involving GPs in joint working. GPs were described as a 'weak professional link in the collaborative chain' (Hudson *et al.*, 1998: 15); the professional culture of general practice 'has not been one of collaboration' (Callaghan *et al.*, 2000: 25).

Both the lack of a collaborative culture and the narrow, practice and patient focus of traditional GP perspectives were apparent in the total purchasing pilot (TPP) schemes – an extension of GP fund-holding in the mid-1990s which offered very considerable budgetary flexibility. Although about a third of TPPs expressed particular interest in purchasing community and continuing care services, they were slow to engage in broader strategic planning activities with social services counterparts (Myles *et al.*, 1998). TPPs also tended to adopt a 'macho' purchasing style, which was not conducive to the development of shared understandings, aims and objectives, or to collaboration in achieving those objectives (Abbott, 1998). Even within the government of the day, there was some concern as to whether this purchasing style, based on 'stand-off' relationships between purchasers and providers, could be effective (Mawhinney, cited in Hudson, 1999). Most significantly, from the point of view of this article, the collaborative vision of GPs involved in TPP and other GP fund-holding schemes largely extended only as far as the purchasing of additional social work services to relieve pressures on their practices (North and Peckham, 2001). This narrow, practice-focused approach led to inequities between groups of patients, which were of considerable concern to local authority partners who saw themselves as responsible for ensuring equitable access to services across the authority as a whole (see, e.g., Bosanquet *et al.*, 1998).

Nevertheless, both before and after the creation of PCG/Ts there have been numerous projects in which social work and other advice and information services have been located in primary care settings. Evaluations of these initiatives have demonstrated positive outcomes, especially improvements in understanding and communication between the professionals involved and in the ease and speed with which patients can obtain services (see Glendinning *et al.*, 1998; Rummery and Glendinning, 2000; Clarke *et al.*, 2001). Despite these successes, such practice-level initiatives were nevertheless difficult to sustain, as prior to the creation of PCG/Ts there was no organisational, funding or commissioning framework by which successful projects could be rolled out. Indeed, the fragmented structure and individualistic focus of general practice meant that such initiatives were not necessarily even located in areas where they might be most needed, but simply where enterprising GP staff happened to negotiate successfully with a local social services agency. Of course, these issues of equity and consistency have not been fully resolved with the creation of PCG/Ts, particularly in larger authorities such as county councils, which may contain several primary care organisations (DH, 1999b).

Progress in Strategic and Operational Collaboration

Some of these historical tensions and difficulties have been echoed in the progress made by PCG/Ts between 1999 and 2002 in developing relationships with local authority partners. The social services representatives initially on PCG boards and now on PCT PECs have typically been senior managers within their own departments, with responsibilities for both service commissioning and operational management. They have thus been ideally placed to liaise with their own departments on both strategic and operational issues. However, this seniority and influence is generally not reflected in their position on PCG boards and PCT PECs, where a declining minority have held any formal office. PCG/T chief officers have also confirmed that social services representatives are less likely to have influence over board decisions than most other categories of members. In 2000, in only 18 per cent of PCG/Ts were social services representatives considered to have great or very great influence in 2000, compared with 64 per cent of PCG/Ts in which GPs were considered to exercise (very) great influence.

Although social services representatives are likely to be crucially important partners in developing services that could prevent hospital admission and support prompt discharge, they appear to remain relatively marginal to most PCG/T service commissioning. By 2002, in the 83 per cent of PCG/Ts with a designated sub-group responsible for service commissioning, less than half (45 per cent) included a social services representative. Wider consultation to inform service commissioning also appeared still to be dominated by medical and nursing perspectives (see Figure 2).

Progress in joint commissioning with local authority social services departments has, however, been rapid, though this largely reflects the priority areas of national NHS modernisation policies. By 2002, many PCG/Ts were commissioning in partnership with social services or other local authority services (Wilkin *et al.*, 2002).

In relation to commissioning older peoples services, by 2002 two-thirds (68 per cent) of PCG/Ts were commissioning community-based rehabilitation schemes jointly with social services, as were 64 per cent for joint assessments, 63 per cent for rapid response home care schemes and 62 per cent for integrated care management.

There is also evidence of efforts to improve collaboration at operational levels. Joint training between groups of NHS and local authority staff was reported to have taken place in 89 per cent of PCG/Ts between 2001 and 2002; this included 'away days' and joint training about the new single assessment process. A similarly high proportion of PCG/Ts reported

FIGURE 2
PERCENTAGES OF COMMISSIONING LEADS RATING STAKEHOLDERS AS
INFLUENTIAL IN COMMISSIONING DECISIONS (2002)

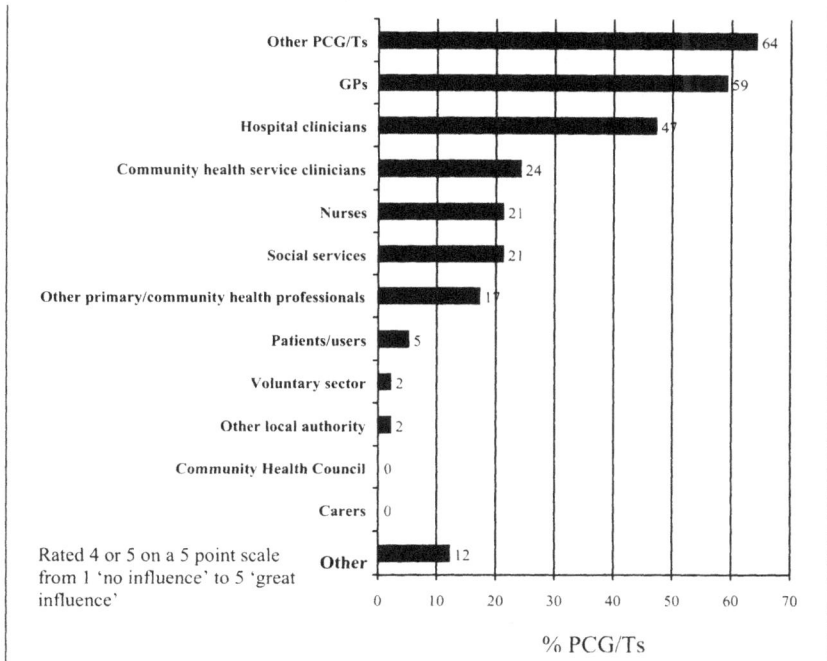

Stakeholder	% PCG/Ts
Other PCG/Ts	64
GPs	59
Hospital clinicians	47
Community health service clinicians	24
Nurses	21
Social services	21
Other primary/community health professionals	17
Patients/users	5
Voluntary sector	2
Other local authority	2
Community Health Council	0
Carers	0
Other	12

Rated 4 or 5 on a 5 point scale from 1 'no influence' to 5 'great influence'

% PCG/Ts

changes in the organisation of front-line health and social care staff over the same period. These changes included the reorganisation of staff teams, secondments, changes in roles and responsibilities and changes in staff terms and conditions of employment (Wilkin *et al.*, 2002). Evidence from the first sites to use the 1999 Health Act flexibilities to create new integrated health and social care services suggests that investment in staff training and similar initiatives may indeed be essential to overcome traditional professional 'tribalisms' and suspicions (Glendinning *et al.*, 2002).

Wider Local Authority Collaborations

Joint commissioning and the integration of health and social services are only part of the potential full range of collaborative relationships between PCG/Ts and local authorities. Working together with local authority partners on the environmental, economic and social factors affecting population health and well-being is also important in relation to PCG/T responsibilities for improving health. Here, the statutory requirement for PCG boards and PCT PECs to include a representative from the local social services department may be a disadvantage. Official guidance on the role of social services representatives suggested that they 'may be able to act as a gateway to other local government departments such as environmental health, housing and education' (NHSE, 1998: para.77). However, differences in the cartographical boundaries of PCG/Ts and local authorities, and divisions of responsibility in areas with two-tier local government structures are both likely to present barriers. Almost half of PCG/Ts were located in areas with two-tier local government structures and in a third of these the population was split between two or more district councils, none of which had rights of representation on the PCG/T Board. By 2002, 24 per cent of PCG/Ts were responsible for patients in local authorities that had no statutory right of representation on their boards, and almost half of both social services representatives and PCG/T chief executives considered that boundary differences created barriers to closer collaboration (Wilkin *et al.*, 2002).

PCG/Ts reported a number of mechanisms for overcoming these problems. In some PCG/Ts, the social services representative had wider responsibilities within her/his authority; this was particularly helpful when it allowed links to be made with the wider community and environmental responsibilities of unitary local authorities. A few PCG/Ts had co-opted additional local authority representatives to their boards or sub-committees. However, most PCG/Ts had established separate, independent relationships with other local authority services and functions, at both district and county levels (Glendinning *et al.*, 2001). When all these mechanisms are taken into account, PCG/Ts' links with other local authority departments over strategic planning, commissioning, operational-level collaboration and health improvement activities are considerable and have clearly increased since 1999 (see Table 1). Moreover, by autumn 2002, all PCG/Ts were involved in local multi-agency partnership initiatives relating to health improvement (see Table 2).

TABLE 1
PCG/T COLLABORATION WITH OTHER LOCAL AUTHORITY DEPARTMENTS (%)

Department	1999 (*n=72*)	2000 (*n=69*)	2002 (*n=66*)
% of PCGs collaborating with:			
Community development /regeneration	58	87	100
Leisure	41	73	80
Education	46	68	76
Housing	47	65	77
Transport	27	54	58
Welfare rights	18	39	35
Special education	13	13	38

TABLE 2
PCG/T INVOLVEMENT IN MULTI-AGENCY INITIATIVES
2000 (N=69) AND 2002 (N=66)

% PCG/Ts	2000	2002
Sure Start	62	85
Better Government for Older People	26	33
New Deal for Communities	22	33
Health Action Zone	23	27
Education Action Zone	17	14

TABLE 3
PCG/T FINANCIAL CONTRIBUTIONS TO NON-NHS INITIATIVES, 2000 (N=69)

% of PCG/Ts	2000	2002
Community development activities	46	76
Leisure/exercise/recreation programmes	46	74
Support for carers	39	72
Accident prevention	28	64
Family support	25	49
Welfare rights advice	32	40
Community transport	13	24

Nevertheless, there are wide variations between PCG/Ts in the scale of these wider collaborative networks. Although by 2002 all PCG/Ts reported involvement in at least one multi-agency collaborative initiative, 21 per cent reported being involved in six or more such collaborations. By 2002, 85 per cent of PCG/Ts reported that they had allocated some resources to a range of health improvement activities (see Table 3). These financial contributions illustrate the flexibility of the budgets for which PCG/Ts are now responsible and the new opportunities for contributing elements of those resources to wider non-NHS functions. Again the extensiveness of these contributions varies widely, but two-thirds (67 per cent) of PCG/Ts were contributing resources to at least three initiatives.

Overall, there is little evidence to suggest that two-tier local authority structures are creating insuperable barriers for PCG/Ts in developing direct links with other local government functions. Indeed, it may be that the PCG/Ts in these areas have invested more effort in developing links with services located at district council level than with those based in the authority from which the social services representative comes, precisely because of the absence of any automatic representation.

In summary, for these new organisations with very substantial responsibilities for managing and developing local NHS services, the creation within three years of such an extensive range of links with social services and other local government functions is undoubtedly a major achievement. However, these collaborative links need to be seen as only the start of a process of collaborative investment, planning and operational development which may take some time to translate into new patterns of services and ways of delivering them. Moreover, a number of other factors within the NHS may impede or divert PCTs from their collaborative agenda. These are discussed below.

The Dominance of GPs

As Lewis (2001: 353) points out, 'the choice of primary care and GPs as the people to make responsible for integrating provision ... is at once logical and surprising'. In numerical terms, general practice perspectives dominated the early PCG boards. In autumn 2000, 91 per cent of Chairs rated GPs' views and interests as well-represented on the PCG Board – an increase from 76 per cent the previous year – compared with 65 per cent who rated social services' views as well represented, 64 per cent rating primary and community nurses' views and interests as well represented and only 30 per cent who rated local public interests as well represented.

This professional hegemony inevitably creates tensions. A third (38 per cent) of social services representatives on the early PCG boards said that the priority accorded to matters of concern to GPs, such as clinical treatments and prescribing, and the dominance of medical culture and service models, constituted continuing obstacles to collaboration. Similarly, it was perhaps not surprising that the flexibilities offered by PCGs' newly unified budgets led, at least initially, to the movement of resources described above towards areas of direct relevance to general practice such as prescribing and practice infrastructure.

Moreover, as Lewis (2001) argues, notions of 'need' and 'care' are materially and conceptually different from concepts of 'illness' and 'treatment'. If these differences are not fully recognised and understood, problems may arise from the inappropriate application of medical models to broader objectives that encompass social inclusion, quality of life and well-being. In this context, strategies for achieving wider social objectives such as maintaining independence, improving health or reducing social exclusion may be marginalised, or reduced to discrete interventions which can be designed and delivered within a 'treatment' paradigm, rather than encompassing broader, more diffuse interventions whose outcomes may be harder to measure and take longer to detect. Initiatives designed to prevent ill-health or slow down a deteriorating condition, where immediate beneficial outcomes are difficult to detect, may be particularly vulnerable.

Since their creation in 1999, it is arguable that the professional hegemony of general practice over the culture, priorities and operations of

PCG/Ts has waned considerably. The abolition of health authorities in 2002 and the rapid transition to Trust status for the remaining PCGs, in order to take over devolved functions from the health authorities, has had a marked impact on their organisational form and modes of operating. The political and policy rhetoric of NHS 'modernisation' refers repeatedly to the strengthened decision-making powers of front-line NHS staff. However, in reality, the increased responsibilities, powers and freedoms that have been devolved to the front-line professionals involved in PCT professional executive committees are tightly circumscribed and subject to an extensive array of targets, standards and inspection systems. The new functions of PCTs – especially their responsibilities for very considerable areas of public expenditure – have therefore been accompanied by substantial new responsibilities and accountabilities on behalf of the professionals who work within, and govern, them (Dowling and Glendinning, 2003). These responsibilities also have the potential to impact on PCTs collaborative capacity.

The Impact of the Drive to 'Modernise'

The 1997 NHS White Paper (Secretary of State, 1997), the NHS Plan (NHS, 2000) and a series of national service frameworks are among a number of measures that have together set national priorities and targets for service development and increased the scrutiny to which the performance of PCTs is subject. These targets include the requirement to collaborate with external partner organisations, and the threat that collaborative mechanisms will be externally imposed on PCTs and local authorities whose performance in this respect is judged to be inadequate. This is not new, but an intensification of the drive to exercise managerial pressure and influence in primary care which arguably began in the early 1990s (Glendinning, 1998; North and Peckham, 2001).

Paradoxically, however, this intensive and urgent NHS 'modernisation' imperative presents some major threats to collaboration with local authority partners (Clarke and Glendinning, 2002). First, a tightly specified, centrally imposed service development agenda has undoubtedly made it difficult for local partnerships to develop their own 'core business' that reflects local priorities and enjoys widespread local ownership. Thus by early 2002, when almost half of our sample of PCGs had already become free-standing Trusts and the remainder were preparing to do so, the social services representatives on their boards reported a range of barriers to collaboration that reflected the rapid and intensive organisational development programme to which PCG/Ts were subject. These problems included lack of time and the pace of change (35 per cent of social services representatives); and the lack of organisational capacity for inter-agency collaboration (15 per cent) (Wilkin *et al.*, 2002).

Collaborative relationships also risk being undermined by accountability and performance management systems that do not allow the 'rewards' of collaboration to be equally distributed between partners. For example, the imperative, repeated in a range of policy documents, to develop new short-term pre-admission and post-discharge services that can prevent hospitalisation and expedite discharge (DH, 2001d) is likely to be of more interest and significance to PCTs and other NHS Trusts than to local authority partners. In contrast, robust and effective partnerships require equal status between partners and fairness in the distribution of partnership benefits and gains (Hudson and Hardy, 2002).

Finally, the very heavy emphasis on the management and measurement of performance in the drive to modernise may undermine local partnerships. Performance indicators and regulatory systems remain largely structured around discrete service or departmental boundaries, rather than being multi-organisational or system-wide (Clarke and Glendinning, 2002). Even localities which have used the flexibilities in the 1999 Health Act to pool NHS and local authority budgets report still having to disaggregate their performance data and account separately for the 'health' and 'social' care elements (Glendinning et al., 2002). It is indeed difficult to measure the outcomes of collaborative, inter-agency activities (Glendinning, 2002), so these are consequently likely to receive less attention from organisations already facing a heavy development agenda. PCG/Ts' plans for future organisational development and change have therefore tended to reflect the dominance of mono-organisational, rather than broader collaborative, objectives and pressures. When asked about their main reasons for becoming Trusts, only 18 per cent of PCGs mentioned the opportunity to develop closer integration of health and social services, compared with 77 per cent who hoped to be able to integrate primary and community health services. The extensive waves of mergers between the original 481 PCGs, particularly during the course of their transition to trust status, were also likely to be prompted by perceived opportunities to enhance organisational capacity to achieve NHS goals and objectives than by a desire to build the conditions for successful collaboration (Wilkin et al., 2002). The prioritisation of NHS modernisation objectives over local collaborations in prompting these rapid organisational developments may be damaging enough; but they also risk disrupting established inter-agency and inter-professional relationships (Hiscock and Pearson, 1999). In contrast, robust partnerships depend to some extent on continuity and commitment among senior personnel, so that shared values and objectives can develop and be sustained (Hudson and Hardy, 2002).

Collaborations between PCG/Ts and local authorities aimed at enhancing individual or community responsibility for health, improving the conditions which affect health or reducing social exclusion are also vulnerable within this enhanced regulatory regime. The potentially perverse effects of focusing organisational attention on what can be measured, combined with incentives to demonstrate success and sanctions in the event of failure, mean that broader health improvement collaborations are at risk of being squeezed out of the partnership agenda (Clarke and Glendinning, 2002). This risk is enhanced by the widespread lack of consensus on appropriate targets, outcome measures and performance indicators; the complexity of interventions that can address multiple causes of inequality (including age, gender and ethnicity as well as socio-economic status); and the long-term nature of any improvements in health status that may result from broad, public health collaborations (Peckham, 2003).

CONCLUSIONS

The measures introduced in England since 1997 to facilitate, encourage and ultimately enforce collaboration, are both extensive and thorough. Unlike previous attempts to promote collaboration, they have the potential to penetrate the 'core business' of NHS and local authority organisations. From the NHS perspective, PCTs constitute a new organisational vehicle within which previously fragmented GP practice-based services can be brought together with community health services and both can be aligned, planned, funded and delivered alongside social and other local authority services. In addition, PCT responsibilities for health improvement as well as health services demand a broad perspective on the health needs of the local population as a whole and collaboration with a wide range of local authority, voluntary and community organisations if these responsibilities are to be effectively discharged. The relocation of public health expertise within PCTs following the abolition of health authorities will undoubtedly assist in the execution of this responsibility.

However, other pressures are likely to impede collaborative developments and could even undermine them. The dominant position of GPs within the early histories of PCGs brought to the fore a historical lack of collaborative involvement, traditional individualistic culture and the legacies of fund-holder type of purchasing styles. All of these are difficult to reconcile with broader collaborative activities. More pervasively, the relentless pursuit by central government of the public sector 'modernisation' enterprise, with its intensification of targets, regulatory frameworks and performance management regimes, risks destabilising, undermining or otherwise seriously damaging local collaborations. Strong and effective partnerships with other agencies and services need a degree of local ownership that may be difficult to sustain in the face of strengthened national targets and 'upwards' accountabilities to central government.

NOTES

1. This article discusses research findings that cover the period from when PCGs were established in 1999, through their gradual transition to PCT status. The first PCGs became PCTs in 2000 and all had become PCTs by April 2003. The initials PCGs\Ts are used as a generic term in this article to cover research findings that apply to both.
2. The English White Paper was followed by similar proposals for the other countries in the UK. Because of the potential for divergence following devolution, this article will concentrate only on the prospects for collaboration in England.

REFERENCES

Abbott, S., 1998, *Total Purchasing at Castlefields: A Case Study*, Report 98/40, Liverpool, Health and Community Care Research Unit.

Abbott, S. and S. Gillham, 2000, 'Health Without a Care', *Health Services Journal*, 2 Nov., p.32.

Audit Commission, 1986, *Making a Reality of Community Care* (London: HMSO).

Bosanquet, N. *et al.*, 1998, *The Bromsgrove Total Purchasing Project 1994–1996* (London: Department of Primary Health and General Practice, Imperial College School of Medicine at St Mary's).

Callaghan, G., M. Exworthy, B. Hudson and S. Peckham, 2000, 'Prospects for Collaboration in Primary Care: Relationships between Social Services and the New PCGs', *Journal of Interprofessional Care*, 14/1, pp.19–26.

Campbell, S. and M. Roland, 2003, 'Improving the Quality of Healthcare through Clinical Governance', in Dowling and Glendinning, 2003.

Clarke, K., S. Sarre, C. Glendinning and J. Datta, 2001, *FWA's WellFamily Service: Evaluation Report* (Manchester: NPCRDC and Department of Applied Social Sciences and London, FWA).

Clarke, J. and C. Glendinning, 2002, 'Partnership and the Remaking of Welfare Governance', in C. Glendinning, M. Powell and K. Rummery (eds.), *Partnerships, New Labour and the Governance of Welfare* (Bristol: Policy Press).

Coleman, A. and C. Glendinning, forthcoming, 'Local Authority Scrutiny of Health: Making the Views of the Community Count?' *Health Expectations*.

Croxon, B., B. Ferguson and J. Keen, 2003, 'The New Institutional Structures: Risks to the Doctor–Patient Relationship', in Dowling and Glendinning, 2003.

Department of the Environment, Transportation and the Regions (DETR), 2001, *Local Strategic Partnerships – Government Guidance* (London: DETR).

DH, 1998, *Modernising Health and Social Services; National Priorities Guidance 1999/00-2001/2* (London: Department of Health).

DH, 1999a, *Saving Lives: Our Healthier Nation* (London: The Stationery Office).

DH, 1999b, *Working in Partnership; Joint Working between Health and Social Services in Primary Care Groups*, Summary of Key Themes from Regional Seminars (London: Joint Unit, Department of Health).

DH, 2000, *Joint Investment Plans*, Health and Social Care Joint Unit, Department of Health, www.doh.gov.uk/joint, 12 Jan.

DH, 2001a, *Health Improvement and Modernisation Plans: Requirements for 2002*, Department of Health, www.doh.gov.uk/himp/himpguid02.pdf.

DH, 2001b, *National Service Framework for Older People* (London: Department of Health).

DH, 2001c, *Care Trusts; Emerging Framework*, www.doh.gov.uk/caretrusts, 14 March.

DH, 2001d, *Intermediate Care*, HSC 2001/01: LAC (2001)1 (London: Department of Health).

DH, 2002, *Involving Patients and the Public in Healthcare: Response to the Listening Exercise* (London: Department of Health).

Dowling B. and C. Glendinning (eds.), 2003, *The New Primary Care: Modern, Dependable, Successful?* (Maidenhead: Open University Press).

Dowling, B. and C. Glendinning, 2003, 'The "New" Primary Care: Ideology and Performance', in Dowling and Glendinning, 2003.

Dowling, B., D. Wilkin and K. Smith, 2003, 'Organisational Development and Governance of Primary Care', in Dowling and Glendinning, 2003.

Dunleavy, A., 1995, 'Policy Disasters: Explaining the UK's Record', *Public Policy and Administration*, 10/2, pp.52–70.

Glendinning, C., 1998, 'From General Practice to Primary Care: Developments in Primary Health Services 1990–1998', in E. Brunsdon, H. Dean and R. Woods (eds.), *Social Policy Review 10* (London: SPA and London Guildhall University).

Glendinning, C., 2002, 'Partnerships between Health and Social Services: Developing a Framework for Evaluation', *Policy and Politics*, 30/1, pp.115–27.

Glendinning, C., K. Rummery and R. Clarke, 1998, 'From Collaboration to Commissioning: Developing Relationships between Primary Health and Social Services', *British Medical Journal*, 317, pp.12–15.

Glendinning, C., S. Abbott and A. Coleman, 2001, '"Bridging the Gap": New Relationships between Primary Care Groups and Local Authorities', *Social Policy and Administration*, 35/4, pp.411–25.

Glendinning, C., B. Hudson, B. Hardy and R. Young, 2002, *National Evaluation of Notifications for Use of the Section 31 Partnership Flexibilities in the Health Act 2002; Final Project Report* (Leeds: Nuffield Institute for Health; Manchester: National Primary Care Research and Development Centre).

Goodwin, N., 2001, 'The Long-Term Importance of English Primary Care Groups for Integration in Primary Heath Care and Deinstitutionalisation of Hospital Care', *International Journal of Integrated Care*, 1/2, pp.1–13.

Guardian Society Supplement, 2003, 14 May, p.5.

Ham, C., 1999, *Health Policy in Britain* (Basingstoke: Macmillan).

HSC, 1998, *The New NHS: Modern, Dependable. Guidance on Health Authority and Primary Care Group Allocations*, Health Service Circular 1998/171 (Leeds: NHS Executive).

Hiscock, J. and M. Pearson, 1999, 'Looking Inwards, Looking Outwards: Dismantling the "Berlin Wall" between Health and Social Services?' *Social Policy and Administration*, 33/2, pp.150–63.

Hudson, B., H. Lewis, E. Waddington and G. Wistow, 1998, *The Interface between Social Care and Primary Care: National Mapping Exercise* (Leeds: Nuffield Institute for Health).

Hudson, B., 1999, Developments at the Health–Social Care Interface', in H. Dean and R. Woods (eds.), *Social Policy Review 11* (Luton: Social Policy Association).

Hudson, B. and B. Hardy, 2002, What Makes a 'Successful' Partnership and How can it be Measured?' in C. Glendinning, M. Powell and K. Rummery (eds.), *Partnerships, New Labour and the Governance of Welfare* (Bristol: The Policy Press).

Iliffe, S., 2001, 'The National Plan for Britain's National Health Service: Towards a Managed Market', *International Journal of Health Services*, 31/1, pp.105–11.

Leutz, W., 1999, 'Five Laws for Integration Medical and Social Services: Lessons from the United States and United Kingdom', *The Millbank Quarterly*, 77/1, pp.77–110.

Lewis, J., 2001, 'Older People and the Health–Social Care Boundary in the UK: Half a Century of Hidden Policy Conflict', *Social Policy and Administration*, 35/4, pp.343–59.

Myles, S. *et al.*, 1998, *Total Purchasing and Community and Continuing Care: Lessons for Future Policy Development in the NHS* (London: Kings Fund).

Newman, J., 2001, *Modernising Governance. New Labour, Policy and Society* (London: Sage).

NHSE, 1998, 'The New NHS. Modern, Dependable. Developing Primary Care Groups', Local Authority Circular LAC(98)21 (Leeds: NHS Executive).

NHS, 2000, *The NHS Plan: A Plan for Investment, a Plan for Reform*, Cm 4818-1 (London: The Stationery Office).

Nocon, A., 1994, *Collaboration in Community Care* (Sunderland: Business Education Publishers).

North, N. and S. Peckham, 2001, 'Analysing Structural Interests in Primary Care Groups', *Social Policy and Administration*, 35/4, pp.426–40.

Paton, C., 1999, 'New Labour's Health Policy', in M. Powell (ed.), New Labour, New Welfare State (Bristol: The Policy Press).

Peckham, S., 2003, 'Improving Local Health', in Dowling and Glendinning, 2003.

Rummery, K. and C. Glendinning, 2000, *Primary Care and Social Services: Developing New Partnerships for Older People* (Oxford: Radcliffe Medical Press).

Secretary of State for Health, 1997, *The New NHS. Modern. Dependable* (London: The Stationery Office).

Secretary of State for Health, 1999, *Saving Lives: Our Healthier Nation* (London: The Stationery Office).

Secretary of State for Health, 2002, *Delivering the NHS Plan: Next Steps on Investment; Next Steps on Reform*, Cm 5503 (London: The Stationery Office).

Walby, S. and J. Greenwell, 1994, 'Managing the National Health Service', in J. Clarke, A. Cochrane and E. McLaughlin (eds.), *Managing Social Policy* (London: Sage).

Wilkin, D., S. Gillham and B. Leese, 2000, *The National Tracker Survey of Primary Care Groups and Trusts: Progress and Challenges 1999/2000* (Manchester: National Primary Care Research and Development Centre).

Wilkin, D., S. Gillham and A. Coleman, 2001, *The National Tracker Survey of Primary Care Groups and Trusts 2000/2001: Modernising the NHS?* (Manchester: National Primary Care Research and Development Centre).

Wilkin, D., A. Coleman, B. Dowling and K. Smith, 2002, *The National Tracker Survey of Primary Care Groups and Trusts 2001/2002: Taking Responsibility?* (Manchester: National Primary Care Research and Development Centre).

Health and Local Government Partnerships: The Local Government Policy Context

STEPHANIE SNAPE

LOCAL GOVERNMENT AND HEALTH

'Short horizons' is one of the chronic afflictions of the public services and its commentators in the United Kingdom. Such short horizons have contributed to a view that the 'traditional' boundary between health services and local government is that of the health–social care divide. However, this 'boundary' has only been in existence in its present form for 30 years (and has constantly been subject to change during this period). Before this, local authorities had a greater role in health service provision. Indeed, from the mid-nineteenth century until at least the creation of the National Health Service, local government was the predominant provider of public health services. Local authorities worked to secure sanitary public health, through the development of healthy water supplies, sewerage, council housing and slum clearance, and refuse collection and waste disposal services. They appointed Medical Officers of Health to assess local health needs. And by the 1930s they were managing a wide range of acute and primary care services, including major hospitals. Indeed, Webster writes that local authorities had by 1939 'assembled a formidable array of specialist health services' and that services had expanded 'to such a degree that this system was already occasionally called a "National Health Service"' (1988: 6–8).[1]

However, by the mid-1970s this pivotal role for local government in healthcare and health policy had been considerably weakened. In 1974 government transferred a number of key local government health services to newly created area health authorities; services which included home nursing, family planning, health education, ambulance services and school health. Medical Officers of Health were also transferred to the NHS and local authorities no longer reported on the health needs of their local area. There is a widely held view that the transferred Medical Officers of Health (since re-titled directors of public health) rapidly became subsumed within the predominant medical model of health within the NHS (Holland and Stewart, 1998; Hunter, 1999). This is highly significant given that the role of Medical Officers of Health was crucial in both providing a conceptual role for local government in health through the concept of 'public health' and a senior officer whose work ensured that health issues remained central to local government.

The 1974 reorganisation is often viewed as a watershed in local government's relationship with health. The 'orthodox' view of the 1974 changes is that it largely transferred local government's involvement in health 'en bloc' to the NHS. And what remained – rather oddly – were local government's welfare services (now termed social services). Today this equates to a range of care and protection services such as residential care homes and day centres for the elderly, drug or alcohol abuse programmes, child protection and fostering, adoption and children's homes for children in care. And the health–social care divide became enshrined as the key boundary between the NHS and local government: the arena in which the two leviathans had to co-operate to provide services to client groups such as the elderly. However, local government actually retained control over major public health services such as housing, leisure services, sanitation and so on. In reality, these services have a greater influence over health and well-being than most NHS services, as Campbell argues:

> Refuse collectors are not highly paid, glamorous figures like brain and heart surgeons, but they almost certainly do more to keep the population healthy than these stars of the health world. Landlords in the largely-unregulated private rented sector are no longer held up as targets for vilification by the media, but they, as well as the length of hospital waiting lists, may sometimes make a contribution to keeping poor people unhealthy. Conversely, research suggests that central heating and insulation improvements to council housing can bring about immediate improvement in respiratory symptoms in children with asthma and a reduction of lost school days...These and many other areas of everyday life that have a huge impact on public health are actually and potentially directly influenced by the work of local authorities. (Campbell, 2000: 13)

Indeed, it is one of the greatest ironies of the modern state that while local government has more influence over the health and well-being of its communities than the NHS, for the last 30 years it has had little influence over the shape of local health policy or the operation of local NHS services. This in itself partly reflects the way in which the NHS has captured and monopolised the public's perception of health; as health and the NHS are often viewed almost interchangeably, with little understanding of the importance of the wider determinants of health and local government's role in shaping these. And, over the years since 1974, many local authority councillors and senior officers simply 'forgot' local government traditions in health and overlooked the council's key role in shaping the health of its communities. The links between housing and health, for example, which were reviewed frequently in the annual reports of the Medical Officers of Health, became less apparent and less the focus of attention either at the corporate centre or when shaping service delivery. Instead, the prevailing interpretation of local government's role in health was one almost totally equating to the health–social care divide.

However, more recent policy developments have provided substantive opportunities for local government to 'revisit' their role in health:

> the new policy context provides opportunities for local authorities to reclaim their original role as champions of the health of local communities ... Promoting the health and well being of local people is at the heart of community leadership. While the NHS has a critical role in our local communities, it is only through real partnerships between the NHS and local government that we can effectively tackle the wider causes of ill health. (SOLACE, 2001: 2)

From an NHS perspective, the post-1997 emphasis within the NHS on tackling health inequalities and addressing the wider determinants of health can be traced back to the 1980 Black Report and the emergence of the 'new public health' movement. Further support for the social model of health was provided by the Acheson report (1998), which clearly demonstrated the highly unequal experiences of ill-health between different socio-economic groups, ethnic groups and gender. The Acheson report also provided the backbone to the new administration's Green Paper on public health, *Our Healthier Nation* (1998). This appeared to demonstrate New Labour's commitment to the values of the new public health movement. However, the publication of *The NHS Plan* was viewed by many as a return to the more 'traditional' focus on the healthcare system and individual lifestyle factors (Hunter, 2000). And certainly there have been examples of contradictions within New Labour health policy; Campbell labels this as 'schizophrenia', as the government emphasises both the broader, societal determinants of health while retaining individualised notions of responsibility for ill health and medically focused targets (2000: 15).

As in the NHS, there were signs prior to 1997 of some local authorities (and departments within authorities) exploring a broader role in health improvement and tackling health inequalities. The new public health movement had influence over some authorities; indeed, it was local government, rather than the NHS, that drove the Healthy City movement in the UK. Experience in developing area regeneration programmes, anti-poverty strategies and Local Agenda 21 also encouraged the realisation of a broader role. However, as with the NHS, New Labour gaining power in 1997 provided a more propitious national policy environment for authorities determined to reclaim their role in health.

Post-1997 there are three key policy areas which could support change in local government's involvement in health: innovations in the health–social care boundary; the 'core' Local Government Modernisation initiatives; and area-based initiatives. There have been substantive policy changes to the health–social care boundary, with central government encouraging local authorities and NHS organisations to work together more closely through the use of pooled budgets, lead commissioning and integrated management systems. In terms of the 'core' Local Government Modernisation initiatives, commentators have in particular stressed the potential of the community leadership role, supported by the new power of well-being, and the health scrutiny role to provide a lever for local authorities wishing to take a broader role in ensuring the good health and well-being of their communities (INLOGOV, 2000; SOLACE, 2001; Campbell, 2000). Finally, since 1997 central government has established a wide range of area-based initiatives, such as Action Zones and New Deal for Communities, which have the potential to re-emphasise the relationship between regeneration and health.

And local authorities have received considerable exhortation and encouragement to use the opportunities provided by this changing health and local government context. The period since 1997 has seen an 'explosion' of interest and policy guidance on local government's role in health, produced by such influential organisations as the Health Development Agency (HDA), Democratic Health Network (DHN), Local Government Association (LGA) and the Society of Local Authority Chief Executives (SOLACE) (Campbell, 2000; LGA, 2000; SOLACE, 2000; Health Select Committee, 2000; Hamer and Easton, 2002; Hamer and Smithies, 2002; Cramp, 2002; HDA, 2003; NHS Confederation, 2003). These organisations have been arguing for local authorities to champion the social model of health by promoting health improvement and tackling health inequalities.

Such a changing policy context – and ample encouragement – would appear to be conducive to local authorities re-imagining their involvement in health. However, is there any evidence for such a fundamental change? This article is drawn from the findings of a desk-based review intended to provide answers to this question. Evidence from the review is presented in the following sections: first, the crucial issue of 'models of health' is examined; this is followed by presentation of an 'ideal type' for a broader role for councils; the next three sections each examine the impact of changes to the health–social care boundary, the 'core' Local Government Modernisation initiatives and the emergence of area-based initiatives respectively. The last section presents the conclusions.

The article argues that assessment of developments in the selected key areas finds that in practice the health–social care boundary remains a dominant presence in local government's vision of health. There has been no paradigm shift in local government's relationship with health. Although progress has been made in the relationship between regeneration and health, and elements of the Local Government Modernisation Agenda hold the potential for more radical change, the primacy of the social care boundary casts a long shadow. Within social care there is again the potential for change but little radical change has been effected. Certainly, local government practice is far removed from the 'ideal type' of a reclaimed pivotal role in local health policy set out in the article. The performance management framework for both sectors is identified as the key obstacle to more radical progress.[2]

MODELS OF HEALTH

Central to the debate over the relationship between local government and health is the issue of 'what is health?' Two interpretations or models of health tend to dominate this debate. The NHS is driven and shaped by the medical model of health. This model sees the NHS focused on the treatment of disease, in which health is defined as the 'absence of disease', symptoms or sickness. The predominance of this model within the NHS has been produced by advances in medical science and the power of the medical profession. Such a model emphasises treatment above prevention; indeed, only one per cent of current NHS expenditure is targeted at prevention schemes (SOLACE, 2001: 2). Consequently, the NHS is often portrayed as an organisation which focuses on 'downstream' issues such as illness and injury.

In contrast, the social model of health recognises the wider determinants of health and seeks to prevent illness and to support well-being and a good quality of life. This model defines health as the outcome of the effects of all the factors shaping the lives of individuals, families and communities. Dahlgren and Whitehead's (1991) representation of the main determinants of health is widely recognised and used as a faithful representation of the range of factors shaping health. In this model, the main determinants of health are represented as different layers of influence. At the centre are the age, sex and constitutional factors shaping health; the next layer comprises individual lifestyle factors, such as exercise patterns; social and community networks also impact upon health; and, finally, the outermost layer represents general socio-economic, cultural and environmental conditions such as work environment, education, housing. Such a model stresses the need to intervene at a number of points; taking action 'upstream' to prevent illness, injury and disability as well as downstream. Commentators tend to perceive local government as the champions of the social model of health (SOLACE, 2001; Campbell, 2000; LGA, 1998).

LOCAL GOVERNMENT AND HEALTH: DEVELOPING A BROADER AGENDA

But what would greater local government involvement in this area actually entail? What would be involved in local authorities developing strategies and initiatives to support well-being? It is relatively easy to determine the general aim of such strategies; they would seek to improve the health and well-being of the population and to address health inequalities. But how?

In 2000, academics at INLOGOV devised 'best practice guidance' for authorities developing local strategies to tackle the wider determinants of ill health (INLOGOV, 2002). This guidance included advice on mainstreaming health, developing a strategic approach, engaging in public consultation, partnerships with other bodies, operational planning and so on. This article partly draws on this earlier work to set out an 'ideal type' of local government engagement in the wider health agenda.

Figure 1 identifies ten components of this ideal type. These ten components cover a variety of issues including information, needs assessment, strategic and operational planning, member and officer roles, and partner and community engagement. They draw on the key benefits that could be produced by broader involvement of local authorities in the health agenda: a commitment to the social model of health, addressing the democratic deficit of the NHS and drawing upon a broader range of skills and competencies. Authorities approaching such an ideal type would truly have reclaimed a more pivotal role in health. However, as will be demonstrated, local government practice in general is far removed from such an ideal type.

THE HEALTH–SOCIAL CARE BOUNDARY

Since the mid-1970s the relationship between local government and the NHS has been dominated by the health–social care boundary. Sullivan and Skelcher have identified three stages in the development of the health–social care relationship (2002: 71–7). In the late 1960s and 1970s there was an emphasis on joint planning and co-ordination of policy development. These attempts at co-ordination have largely been viewed as unsuccessful (Hudson and Henwood, 2002: 155). And so have the developments in the second stage of the 'mixed economy of care', from the 1980s until 1997, where the emphasis on co-ordination was also enjoined by

FIGURE 1
LOCAL GOVERNMENT ENGAGEMENT IN HEALTH: AN IDEAL TYPE

Issue/Factor/Mechanism	Ideal Type/Good Practice
1. **Information**	Common, 'agreed' information and datasets between local government and health documenting quality of life and ill health.
2. **Assessment of health needs**	Joint, collaborative approach to a comprehensive health needs assessment.
3. **Strategic planning**	'Joined up', coherent approach to strategic planning for health and other key cross-cutting issues across the local government and NHS sectors.
4. **Operational planning and delivery**	Innovative and creative approaches to collaboration in the detail of operational planning and delivery, to include full 'take-up' of the freedoms and flexibilities now on offer to local government and NHS
5. **Mainstreaming health issues**	Health improvement, well-being and tackling inequalities in health to be viewed as a key strategic priority within the local authority
6. **Political leadership and engagement**	Clear political leadership for health issues, through the appointment of a cabinet post for health. All councillors to view health as key strategic priority. Active health scrutiny function.
7. **Officer leadership and engagement**	Health to be seen as a key corporate issue within the senior management team. All departments to be aware of their contribution to good and poor health. Health also to be viewed as local government priority within all tiers of local government employees.
8. **Wide 'partner' engagement**	Other public, private and third sector 'partners' to be engaged in the council's work on health
9. **Community engagement**	Council to actively engage their communities, through a range of mechanisms, in their work on health
10. **Regenerating local communities**	Councils to pursue neighbourhood, area-based initiatives, for communities with poor health

exhortation to involve a range of other public, private and third sector providers through quasi markets for health and community care.

Sullivan and Skelcher's third phase is that of 'strategic collaboration'. They argue that since 1997 New Labour has 'overlaid' the continuing purchaser–provider split with an emphasis on cross-sectoral collaboration

FIGURE 2
KEY PARTNERSHIP INITIATIVES BETWEEN HEALTH AND
SOCIAL CARE SINCE 1997

Initiative	Key Partnership Features
Primary Care Groups/ (PCG/Ts)	Initiative proposed in NHS White Paper, *New NHS, Modern, Trusts Dependable* (1997). PCTs expected to work closely with social services on planning and delivery of services. PCT boards to include social services membership.
S.29–31 Health Act 1999	Initially outlined in *Partnership in Action* (DoH, 1998). S.29 expanded the ability of the NHS to fund local authority work related to health. S.30 created a reciprocal power to fund transfers from local government to health. S.31 introduced three 'flexibilities': pooled budgets; lead commissioning; and integrated provision.
Duty of Partnership	NHS bodies and local authorities required to 'work together for the common good'.
Health Improvement and Modernisation Plans	HIMPs are local strategies for improving health and health care and delivering better integrated care. They are also the means to deliver national targets in each health authority area. Health authorities have lead responsibility but the process should be interagency.
Joint Health and Social Services Appointments Public Health	First proposed in White Paper, *New NHS, Modern, Dependable* (1997). Encouragement of local authority participation in health authority planning activities, and reciprocal arrangements for Directors of Public Health to attend relevant meetings of the local authority. Included within Green Paper, *Our Healthier Nation* (DoH, 1998) and White Paper, *Saving Lives* (DoH, 1999).
Health Action Zones	Pilot projects using interagency partnerships to improve health and relevant services. Targeted at areas of greatest deprivation and inequalities in health.
Promoting Independence Partnership Grant	Included within White Paper, *Modernising Social Services* (DoH, 1998), grant of £647 m to 'foster partnership between health and social services'. Success in obtaining funds depends upon good joint working.
Joint Investment Plans	NHS bodies and local authorities to review and plan together, services for frail older and disabled people.
Joint National Priorities Guidance	National Priorities Guidance set out for both the NHS and social services since 1998. Social services lead on children's welfare, regulation and interagency working. Health lead on waiting lists/times, primary care, coronary heart disease and cancer. 'Shared lead' on cutting health inequalities, mental health and promoting independence.

FIGURE 2 (cont.)

Initiative	Key Partnership Features
Joint National Service Frameworks (NSFs)	Set national standards and define service models for a specific service or care group. First NSFs for coronary heart disease and mental health later followed by NSF for Older People.
Better Government for Older People	Set up in 1997 to improve public services for older people by better meeting their needs, listening to their views and encouraging and recognising their contribution. Chaired by Cabinet Office, supported by partnership working between central and local government, together with national charities and organised through 28 pilot projects.
Care Trusts	Proposed in the *NHS Plan* (2000). Trusts would provide integrated care for older people and those with mental health problems. First 4 Trusts established April 2002.

Source: Adapted from Hudson and Henwood, 2002: 158, and Campbell, 2000: 17–18.

and partnership. One of the first documents to set out the government's agenda of collaboration was *Partnerships in Action* (DoH, 1998). Its key proposals were enacted as sections 29 to 31 of the 1999 Health Act: section 29 expanded the possibilities for funding transfers from the NHS to local authorities; section 30 created a similar reciprocal relationship for local authority funding of health authorities for certain functions; and section 31 removed legal obstacles to joint working by introducing pooled budgets, lead commissioning and the possibility of creating integrated provider organisations.

There have also been a range of other initiatives which have sought to engender partnership working between health and social care, which are summarised in Figure 2. These include the duty of partnership, the involvement of local government in Health Improvement Programmes (HImPs), later amended to Health Improvement and Modernisation Programmes (HIMPs); developments in public health; health action zones; the Promoting Independence Partnership Grant of £647m included in the Social Services White Paper; Joint Investment Plans; Joint National Priorities Guidance. Hudson and Henwood argue that 'these measures amounted to the first coherent strategy on partnership working in the history of British social policy' (2002: 159).

The partial nature of the available evidence makes it difficult to come to a firm conclusion about the success or failure of this partnership approach. There is some evidence supporting the case for marked progress and success in terms of establishing more collaborative relationships (Hudson *et al.*,

1998; Hudson and Lewis, 1999). In particular, the findings of the LGA (2000) survey on the relationship between health and local government are often quoted. In this survey, 80 per cent of local authority respondents reported a positive relationship with the local health sector and almost 90 per cent believed that their relationship with health had improved since 1997. The Social Services Inspectorate's review of the progress being made by nine councils in implementing the Modernisation Agenda for social care also drew very positive conclusions:

> In all councils there was considerable evidence that partnership working, both in the planning and delivery of services, had developed substantially in recent years. Working corporately with key stakeholders was increasingly the norm and there was little evidence of the 'Berlin Wall' of five years ago. Evidence from this and other national inspections indicated that although some more difficult relationships remain – in areas such as continuing health care criteria or delayed hospital discharge – disagreements were less frequent and more easily resolved. Today, if a wall remains at all it appears largely redundant, breached in many places and now the scene of only border skirmishes. (2002: 19)

The report states that considerable progress had been made in both strategic planning and operational partnerships.

Other sources of evidence are more cautious about progress. The 2001/2 Annual Report of the Social Services Inspectorate and Audit Commission Joint Review Team reports a mixed picture of progress in collaboration with some councils making good progress on joint working, while others were 'still in the throes of achieving the attitudinal changes which are clearly required' (2002: 17). Similarly, the 2001/2 Report of the Chief Inspector of Social Services portrays varying success, both between authorities and across client and service groups. In particular, the Report argues that 'inspection evidence has shown that strategic partnership activity has been established across most adults services but is, as yet, underdeveloped in children's services' (2002: 31). The report was also critical of the progress on the Health Act flexibilities, stating that although in spring 2001 councils reported that 518 initiatives to use the flexibilities were in preparation 'by the Autumn there was little progress to report' (2002: 30).

Despite the above reservations, there do appear to have been considerable changes – and improvements in collaboration – across the health–social care divide. However, these changes have not in general been used by local authorities to lever radical change in the health–local government relationship. Certainly collaboration is now more prevalent along the health–social care boundary but the changes do not equate to local authorities reclaiming their pivotal role in health policy. Instead they represent changes at the margins of the boundary which ensure that the vast majority of councils remain far removed from the ideal type outlined in Figure 1.

THE LOCAL GOVERNMENT MODERNISATION AGENDA

As discussed in the introduction, some commentators have argued that elements of the Local Government Modernisation Agenda such as community leadership and health scrutiny provide key opportunities for councils seeking to broaden their role in health policy. However, these particular components of modernisation should not be examined in isolation; it is important to assess the impact of the full range of Local Government Modernisation initiatives. This article takes the two local government White Papers published since 1997 as key reference points for the 'core' Modernisation Agenda initiatives (DETR, 1998; DTLR, 2001). Three broad areas are examined in depth:

- Community Governance (community leadership, the power of well-being, community strategies and local strategic partnerships);
- Improvement Agenda (Best Value, public service agreements, comprehensive performance assessment, social services star ratings, beacon council scheme, freedoms and flexibilities and capacity building);
- New Council Constitutions (executive and scrutiny arrangements).[3]

Community Governance

- Community Leadership

As Clarke and Stewart argue, 'there has always been a tension between a concept of the role of local authorities as local government with a wide-ranging concern for their area that extended beyond the services provided and a concept of local government as an agency for the delivery of a series of services' (2000: 127). This community leadership versus service delivery debate runs well back into the nineteenth century. Since 1997 New Labour has consistently encouraged local authorities to work to develop the community leadership role. As the first White Paper stated: 'Community leadership is at the heart of the role of modern local government. Councils are the organisations best placed to take a comprehensive overview of the needs and priorities of their local areas and communities and lead the work to meet those needs and priorities in the round' (1998: 79). New Labour's second term White Paper also reaffirmed the importance of strong community leadership (2001). Clarke and Stewart (2000) argue that the key mechanisms for achieving success in this area are the process of community planning and the new power of well-being. Latterly, the work of Local Strategic Partnerships (LSPs) can be added to the above.

It is this renewed governmental interest in community leadership which has fuelled the excitement of organisations such as the Democratic Health Network and the Health Development Agency with the current prospects for local councils reclaiming a more central role in local health policy. Rationally, it is obvious that emphasis on such a broad role for local government in protecting and shaping community well-being would include oversight and involvement in health. However, finding substantive evidence to assess developments in community leadership and their impact on health is highly problematic. The concept itself is somewhat 'blurred' and difficult to define; indeed, it is easier to see community leadership in terms of its component elements, such as engaging communities and working in partnership (which in turn are difficult to define). This means that designing an evaluation framework would be highly problematic. And, certainly, there has been no comprehensive, holistic evaluation of local councils' role as 'community leaders'.

• Power of Well-Being
As stated above, the establishment of a power for local authorities to promote the economic, social and environmental well-being of their communities has been viewed as a key mechanism to develop community leadership and governance. In the original 1999 White Paper, the government was proposing a new 'duty' of well-being, but by the time of the Local Government Act 2000 this had been transformed into a discretionary 'power'. This new power, which came into effect in October 2000, is the closest English local authorities have ever been to working within a 'general competence' legal framework enjoyed by so many of their European counterparts. Although the Act included restrictions on the power and a reserve power for the Secretary of State to create further restrictions, it still represents a broad flexible power; as Clarke and Stewart observe this is 'an important step forward' for English local authorities (2000: 131).

The power enables local authorities to do anything they consider is likely to promote or improve the economic and/or social and/or environmental well-being of their area (or part of their area). It includes the power for local authorities to incur expenditure, provide financial assistance, take on functions currently provided by other organisations, create companies and provide staff, goods, services or accommodation. It is also clear from reading the guidance on the power that government expected it to provide support for local authorities tackling obdurate social problems, including poor health: 'It is also recognised that an integrated approach to improving economic, social and environmental well-being is essential to improving health and reducing inequalities' (DETR, 2001: 8). The importance of health and health inequalities looks likely to have partly shaped one important component of the power: the freedom for councils to take action that affects areas outside their own boundaries if the action contributes to the well-being of their own area. Paragraph 53 of the guidance makes clear the significance of this to the relationship with health:

> This is a key power in relation to local authorities' partnership working with the health sector, since most local authorities are not coterminous with health authorities. The power provides opportunities for action between neighbouring health and local authorities and other sub-regional agencies or services where the health and well-being of certain groups cut across traditional service boundaries: for example, travelling communities, people that live and work/study in different authorities, people in a local authority using health services in another area and so on. It also enables joint action to protect the well-being and health of communities at risk from environmental pollution, crime, economic decline or health hazards when these communities reside across authorities' boundaries. (DETR, 2001: 13)

To date there has been no substantive national evaluation of the uptake and use of the new power, however it is generally perceived within local government that little use has been made of it. Consequently, it is likely that little use – if any – has been made of the power in terms of local government's wider role in health. There are two explanations for such low uptake: first, it could be that local authorities had sufficient legal powers without recourse to this new power – this may apply particularly to health given the Health Act flexibilities; and, second, it may be that almost 30 years of increasingly centralised central–local relations has produced a local government tier that is conditioned to top-down policy prescription and uncertain of using more bottom-up, discretionary, powers.

• Community Strategies

The new duty of community strategies, first outlined in the 1998 White Paper, was included within the Local Government Act 2000. Government Guidance provides the following definition: 'A community strategy should aim to enhance the quality of life of local communities and contribute to the achievement of sustainable development in the UK through action to improve the economic, social and environmental well-being of the area and its inhabitants' (DETR, 2000). The government has not prescribed the content, form or timing of these strategies. However, the expected key components would be a long-term vision for the area focusing on the outcomes to be achieved; an action plan identifying shorter term priorities and activities; a shared commitment – across the partners involved – to implement the action plan and proposals to do so; arrangements for monitoring, review and reporting to communities. Prior to determining the vision for the area, the needs and priorities of the communities involved would have to be assessed. Further, the role of communities and citizens is pivotal, with government expecting community strategies to fundamentally engage local communities in identifying problems, needs and priorities and in shaping the development and delivery of the strategy.

There has been no comprehensive national evaluation of community strategies and much 'evidence' is largely anecdotal and patchy. However, some limited research – drawing on analysis of the community strategies produced by 30 local authorities and case studies of good practice – has been undertaken by the HDA (in partnership with other agencies) examining the links between health and community strategies (Hamer and Easton, 2002; Hamer and Smithies, 2002). Although there is much innovative practice – and practice is developing at a frighteningly fast pace – the general picture is one in which the health–social care boundary dominates. The HDA research found that although health featured 'significantly' in community strategies – which are often shaped around such key wicked issues – that 'the ways in which "health" is described reflects a continuum from health as "health and social care" (the most common definition), though to "health and social regeneration" (the least common)' (Hamer and Easton, 2002: 8).

Further, the review found that: few community strategies explicitly state how the component parts of the strategy contribute to health improvement; 'in many cases no clear approach to health improvement is made explicit beyond health and social care'; health priorities within the strategies tend to be dominated by the joint national priorities; community engagement and consultation in the main does not make explicit their interpretation of health, often leading to 'an assumption that the focus of consultation is on service provision or individual lifestyle issues rather than the determinants of health'; although 'there is evidence of pooling of budgets across health and social care there is very little between health and other local government functions'; and usually the HIMP/HAZ acts as the 'health' component of the strategy, often restricting strategic health planning to 'links between health and social care and a few broader based but short-term projects' (Hamer and Easton, 2002: 8–9). Taken in total, such findings present a general picture of the continuing dominance of the health–social care boundary in community strategies, with a few 'leading edge' authorities bucking this general trend to develop more innovative relationships.

- Local Strategic Partnerships

Local Strategic Partnerships (LSPs) are cross-sectoral umbrella partnerships bringing together the public, private, community and voluntary sectors to provide a single, strategic framework within which other, more specific, partnerships can operate. They have four core tasks: preparing and implementing community strategies; providing a forum for co-ordinating and rationalising a wide range of plans and initiatives; working with councils to devise appropriate targets for Public Service Agreements; developing and delivering a Local Neighbourhood Renewal Strategy (where appropriate).

Evidence on the development of LSPs has been partial to date (LGA, 2002: ODPM, 2002; Russell, 2002). No research – other than the HDA-led research discussed above – has specifically focused on the profile of health issues within LSPs. However, certain key findings from existing studies would appear to be relevant to this discussion. First, it is important to emphasise the early stage of development of LSPs; the relationship and interpretation of health will therefore in many LSPs be in the early stages. This will particularly be the case for LSP areas where there was little history of partnership working. In contrast, in those areas where LSPs are based on substantive previous partnership working, there has been a tendency to develop 'partnership of partnerships' structures; where a range of partnerships nestle within the LSP framework (ODPM, 2002: 18). In this way the Health Improvement and Modernisation Programme (HIMP) could simply be incorporated as the health cluster in the LSP; supporting the evidence provided by the HDA study that the HIMP/HAZ is usually taken as the 'health' component of the community strategy. It may also be significant that PCTs are now expected to drive the HIMP (previously HImP); it could be that PCTs are more likely to adopt a medical model approach than the 'strategic' health authorities which previously oversaw the HImP.

Other key findings from preliminary research include the lack of progress being made by most LSPs in integrating plans, strategies and performance indicators (ODPM, 2002: LGA, 2002). Although research found progress in developing a strategic framework and in consensus building, the degree of plan, partnership and performance integration was low. This was explained by a range of factors including that only local authorities were compelled by statutory duty and the problems faced by dissonance of national and local performance targets. Further, an evaluation of the LGA's New Commitment to Regeneration Pathfinders (precursors of LSPs) found that moving from strategic setting and action planning to delivery was enormously challenging and problematic (Russell, 2002).

Improvement Agenda

• Best Value

The cornerstone of the performance management of local authorities between 1997 and 2002 was the Best Value regime which placed a legal duty on local authorities to 'make arrangements to secure continuous improvement in the way functions are exercised, having regard to a combination of economy, efficiency and effectiveness' (Local Government Act, 1999). The component parts of the Best Value regime are now very familiar: the programme of fundamental reviews; the process of Best Value reviews driven by the four Cs of challenge, comparison, consultation and competition; the annual Best Value Performance Plan; and the national Best Value Performance Indicators (BVPIs).

Although in theory Best Value provides some scope for local authorities to reclaim a more pivotal role in local health policy, in practice the regime has proved to be one of the most obdurate barriers to such a change, for the following reasons:

• *Absence of Strong 'Challenge' Culture.* Local authorities have been weak in developing the 'challenge' element of Best Value; failing to fundamentally question the need for existing services or the need to establish new services – yet the latter in particular might have been a useful tool for authorities in reconsidering their health role;
• *Dominance of Service Best Value Reviews.* The majority of Best Value reviews are of a specific service or a component part of a service. Rarer are the cross-cutting reviews, reviews focused on client groups or on geographical locations. Such a pattern of reviews tends to promote and 'protect' the traditional social care boundary between health and local government.
• *Nature of Best Value Performance Indicators (BVPIs).* The national BVPIs have also been a powerful barrier to more radical work by local authorities on health. Although these national indicators have been amended periodically, they reinforce a service-based model of working, with the vast majority of categories of indicators and the indicators themselves based on services. The main exception is the Corporate Health category. However, the Guidance for the 2003/4 indicators only includes one BVPI relevant to partnership working; BV1, which includes four basic questions on the community strategy. In contrast, the Social Services BVPI category includes a range of service based indicators, capturing service performance in terms of looked after children, reviews of child protection cases, production of care packages and so on. And it is important to note that these BVPIs are drawn from

the Social Services Inspectorate Performance Assessment Framework indicators.

• Local Public Service Agreements (Local PSAs)
A local PSA is a voluntary agreement negotiated between an individual local authority and the government. The overall aim of the programme of local PSAs is to improve the delivery of local services through a greater focus on outcomes. Twenty pilot authorities began the programme in late 2000. Since then a roll-out to all upper tier authorities has started. Each local PSA involves an authority agreeing to achieve a range of ambitious targets. In return, an authority is offered a pump-priming grant, scope for extra borrowing and possible freedoms and flexibilities from statutory and administrative constraints. In the longer run, the financial rewards – through the Performance Reward Grant (PRG) – could be substantial. As stated, participating authorities are expected to select 12 or so targets to work towards. However, the majority must be drawn from the list of national targets. Authorities must select at least one social services and education target. For social services the list of national targets is relatively unsurprising, with the first target relating to hospital discharges. However, there are also two targets relating to inequalities in health.

• Comprehensive Performance Assessment
The second Labour administration has developed another performance management system: the Comprehensive Performance Assessment (CPA). There remains real confusion about how BV and CPA relate to each other, but CPA is currently enjoying a higher profile. The Audit Commission (2002: 1) argues that CPA is unique in providing a 'single framework' which pulls together performance information on councils from a range of sources. There are two elements to the CPA: the corporate assessment of councils' ability to improve; and service performance information relating to seven core services (for all authorities but district councils).

The Corporate Assessment does provide some room for recognising the partnership and community leadership role of councils; indeed, the Audit Commission's distinction between an 'excellent' and a 'good' authority partly rests on the formers greater ability to work in partnership (2002: 3). The Audit Commission has also gone to some length to play up the importance of community leadership within the improvement agenda (see Audit Commission, 2003a; 2003b). However, more than offsetting this is the dominance of the service performance data. For social services this is based on the Social Services Inspectorate Personal Social Services star ratings system (Audit Commission, 2003a: 23–6). These reaffirm the primacy of the traditional social care boundary with health. And, as the

Audit Commission itself admits, its CPA framework does not 'explicitly score council performance in cross-cutting areas' – a rather startling omission! (Audit Commission, 2003a: 34).

• Social Services Star Ratings

In May 2002 the Social Services Inspectorate (SSI) published the first Star Ratings for Social Services Departments. This pools performance information from a variety of sources to provide an overall performance rating from 0 to 3 (SSI, 2002a: 11–18). Performance data is taken from the Performance Assessment Framework (PAF) Indicators and other national data; evidence from SSI inspections and SSI/Audit Commission Joint Reviews; SSI performance monitoring of progress in achieving national objectives and targets; and information from external auditors. Although the SSI argue that one of the key differences between three-star councils and two-star councils lies in the formers ability to work innovatively in partnership, in practice the performance data are not directly capturing partnership capacity or capability but the delivery of largely national service targets. And such targets continue to embrace a largely traditional view of the health–social care boundary. And what is crucial here is how much other performance management systems 'buy-in' the SSI performance indicators and ratings; both BV and CPA rely on these. This works to 'import' the primacy of the social care boundary.

• Beacon Council Scheme

The Beacon Council Scheme was initiated as part of the first Labour administration's approach to driving up service standards. The scheme seeks to identify councils which are providing excellent and innovative services or initiatives in order to encourage the dissemination of good practice. There have now been four annual rounds of the scheme. For each round a number of service and cross-cutting themes are identified. Although the 'usual suspects' from social services are present in themes (such as fostering and independent living for older people) the scheme has also worked to develop a strong cross-cutting approach, including themes on neighbourhood renewal and community cohesion. In particular, Round Two incorporated an innovative theme on councils with effective strategies to tackle the wider causes of ill-health. However, the impact of such voluntary schemes set against the power of performance management systems such as the Star Ratings, BV and CPA has to be limited.

• Freedoms and Flexibilities

Increasingly central government has been linking 'good' performance to 'rewards' in terms of freedoms and flexibilities from statutory and administrative regulations. Government has also promised a lighter touch inspection and audit regime for high performing councils. Such an approach has been a key element of the CPA framework, the local PSA Programme and the Social Services Star Ratings system. It is too early to tell what effect this might have on the partnership agenda in general and the relationship between health and local government in particular. It could be argued that offering greater flexibility might produce more radical innovation. However, it is interesting to note the contents of one of the most recent developments in this area. In June 2003 the prospectus of the Innovation Forum was published (ODPM, 2003). The Forum brings together central government and the 22 authorities categorised as 'excellent' in the CPA process. It intends to work on four prioritised agreed themes; one of these is the issue of hospital discharge. And despite the claims of the prospectus that the Forum will represent national and local priorities, the first four seem largely to cohere with the former rather than the latter.

- Capacity Building

Those councils which are awarded poor performance ratings (either through CPA or through individual service ratings such as the SSI Star Ratings) will receive both capacity building support and an intensified inspection regime. The latter is being referred to by the Audit Commission as 'strategic regulation' (2003a); targeting those councils which require the most intensive inspection 'support'. Central government is also developing a Capacity Building programme to improve the skills and abilities of the members and officers in poor performing authorities. It is intended that this programme will include an element of capacity building for partnership working. As with freedoms and flexibilities, it is too early to determine the impact these developments will have on local authorities and health.

New Council Constitutions

New Labour has fundamentally re-shaped the landscape of political management in local councils. The Local Government Act 2000 forced authorities to adopt one of three executive models, although a 'fourth option' of a streamlined committee system also emerged for district councils. Executive models are based on a split between an executive which takes decisions (within a budget and policy framework set by full council) and overview and scrutiny which holds the executive to account and undertakes a broader role in terms of contributing to policy development and review. The vast majority of councils opted for a cabinet with a leader option, producing at most an executive of ten members. Ten councils have established an elected mayor with cabinet and one an elected mayor with a council manager. And there are 50-plus authorities with a streamlined committee system.

On paper at least this is a radical change from the previous committee system, which involved decentralisation of decision-making through a range of committees and sub-committees. In terms of 'health', most authorities would have argued that such a role was undertaken by the Social Services Committee and sub-committees. In such a system the chair of the committee and director of social services were extremely powerful. However, such committees and their sub-committees also provided for wider involvement of members and co-optees. (Few district councils had established any kind of general 'health' committee prior to new political management arrangements being introduced.)

In terms of the local government's relationship with health, new council constitutions have had an impact in two main areas: executive members and their roles; and the development of health scrutiny. In terms of the 'dominant' executive model of the cabinet and leader, the establishment of cabinets might conceivably have provided an opportunity to radically re-cast council priorities on the basis of political priorities, such as 'healthier communities'. And, there is evidence from the Democratic Health Network that some authorities have developed innovative links between health and environmental health, housing and education through linking health portfolios with these areas (Campbell, 2001). However, this research also found that three-quarters of councils with social services functions that had set up executive and scrutiny bodies, had joined their health portfolio with social services. In this way, the key officer supporting the 'social care and health' cabinet member is likely to be the director of social services. Such a development is not surprising and has the consequence of maintaining the clear equation for those in local councils between health and social care.

In terms of health scrutiny, local councils' role in this area of external scrutiny has been given a legislative basis by the Health and Social Care Act 2001. The Act provided social service authorities with the power to review and scrutinise health service matters. Health scrutiny is one of a range of public and patient involvement mechanisms designed by the government to replace the Community Health Councils. The development of health scrutiny has produced a wealth of good practice guidance (Audit Commission, 2001; HDA, 2003; Hamer, 2003; LGA, 2000b). There also appears to have been some innovative work undertaken by authorities which would support councils taking a broader, more holistic view of their role in health. For example, Hamer quotes a number of scrutiny reviews which address inequalities in health, including Bristol's review of the impact of regeneration initiatives on health inequalities. Certainly, there is the potential for health scrutiny to work to support this broader agenda but will this potential be realised?

There are a number of factors which present considerable barriers. The most important is resources. As yet, the government has not dedicated any resources to support local authorities' work in this area. Given that health scrutiny is a power and not a duty, it is not surprising that a number of social services authorities did not have a health scrutiny system up and running when the powers came on line in January 2003. Further, there are very few powers and sanctions available to authorities exercising this role. Also, health scrutiny sits within a poorly devised and confusing new system for supporting patient and public involvement in the NHS. Lastly, overview and scrutiny is struggling generally in local government (Snape and Taylor, 2001; Snape, 2002; Leach, 2002) and health scrutiny does not appear to be any exception to this general position.

Overall, this analysis of the role of health within the Local Government Modernisation Agenda demonstrates that there is considerable potential for a range of modernisation initiatives to lever more radical change. However, in practice change on the ground has been limited. And the principal reason for this lies in the dissonance between the community governance and democratic renewal agenda on one hand and the improvement agenda on the other. The nature of the improvement agenda reinforces the primacy of the social care boundary and the prioritisation of national service concerns at this boundary, most importantly hospital discharges.

REGENERATION AND HEALTH

The mushrooming of Area Based Initiatives (ABIs) since 1997 has produced New Deal for Communities, the Neighbourhood Renewal Strategy, The LGA's New Commitment to Regeneration and a range of Action Zone initiatives (to name but a few). These have developed from a strong economic regeneration base established by local authorities prior to 1997 through Challenge Funding and latterly Single Regeneration Budget programmes. City Challenge was developed in 1991 and the Single Regeneration Budget Challenge Fund was first created in 1994. Both relied on competitive bidding for regeneration funding in deprived areas.

There has been a general recognition that the thrust of regeneration work has increasingly moved from a bricks and mortar, construction-based approach to more holistic approaches to community regeneration which recognise the complex interplay of economic, social and political forces within a community. Certainly, since 1997 government has worked to ensure that ABIs address the whole range of cross-cutting, wicked issues that impact on deprived communities. This has created a strong relationship between ABIs and the developing social inclusion/exclusion agenda (Newman and Geddes, 2001). Such ABIs also rely heavily on cross-sectoral collaboration between public, private and third sector agencies. And, increasingly, a leading role is assigned to the community itself to guide the priorities, processes and structures of regeneration programmes.

As the nature of regeneration work has broadened to include a focus on tackling a range of cross-cutting wicked issues, the role of health in regeneration has been strengthened. Early evidence to support this was provided by a 1998 survey by the Local Government Association of the work being undertaken by local authorities aimed at tackling health inequalities through social and economic regeneration (LGA, 1998). The study found that 'the integration of the health agenda into the regeneration agenda is striking, with health rarely an add-on or an afterthought ... Local government has clearly made the connection between social inclusion and health inequality, integrating the need to tackle both at the core of the regeneration agenda' (1998: 8).

This strong link between health and regeneration was more recently recognised in central government's work on neighbourhood renewal (Social Exclusion Unit, 2001; Neighbourhood Renewal Unit, 2002). The Neighbourhood Renewal Fund (NRF) and the 88 local authority Neighbourhood Renewal Fund areas work within a strategy which recognises five domains of neighbourhood renewal. These five domains are: employment and economies; crime; education and skills; health; housing and the physical environment. The NRF authorities are undertaking a wide range of work in order to tackle health inequalities in their communities.

So health – and a broad social model of health at that – does feature clearly in regeneration work. Such a trend ensures that a relatively high proportion of authorities working in deprived areas are working to address inequalities in health. However, some important questions remain. One is whether ABIs are really 'mainstreamed' into the corporate governance of these authorities? Or, instead, is such work an 'add-on' which is poorly integrated with other 'mainstream' corporate work? ABIs are concentrated in urban areas with high indices of deprivation. This does seem to produce a strong correlation in these areas between regeneration and tackling health inequalities, but what about other local authorities? And is the link between inequalities and regeneration the only wider definition of health that authorities wish to promote? There are also considerable barriers within these deprived communities to making progress on tackling social exclusion (including poor health), which are well recognised within the extensive regeneration literature.

CONCLUSIONS

To conclude, the social care boundary continues to dominate the local government view of health. There has been no paradigm shift; no early twenty-first century renaissance of local government's previous pivotal role in local health policy. Instead, the primacy of the social care boundary remains largely unbreached. Certainly, some good progress has been made in the field of regeneration and health. However, although there have been changes in the social care field, the evidence is confused about their impact and such developments are largely tinkering at the margins rather than more radical change. Perhaps most disappointingly, the real potential within the Local Government Modernisation Programme – particularly in terms of democratic renewal and community governance – has produced few real innovations in practice. There is also a real 'patchiness' and variation in practice across local authorities. But even given such divergence in practice few authorities can claim to be even approaching the ideal type outlined in Figure 1.

Given the range of levers that authorities could use to develop a more radical, holistic approach to health, why has there been such limited success? The key reason is the barrier provided by the local government and NHS performance management systems. For local government, the current performance management framework is dominated by the social care agenda, and, within this, often by the national priorities being promoted by central government. The 'importing' of the SSI performance system into the BV and CPA process only reaffirms the primacy of the social care boundary. And such frameworks cannot simply be ignored by councils; instead they drive and shape local priorities and actions. After all, financial incentives, freedoms and flexibilities, light touch inspections, good reputations, and political and officer careers rest on being awarded good ratings. Such systems shape behaviour and attitudes. They equate to the 'must dos' on the local agenda, compared to the 'might dos' or 'could dos'.

Another key factor is the importing of the social care agenda into the corporate governance and partnership working of an authority. This is clearly demonstrated in the area of performance management. The analysis above also showed how the social care agenda can become incorporated within new political management structures and community strategies and LSPs. This reflects the dominant culture within local government, which simply equates health to social care (and even more bluntly 'social services'). There will need to be a far more fundamental culture change before this link is really challenged.

However, there is a third issue. It may well be that 20 to 30 years of increasing central control has produced a central–local relationship in which local government largely reacts to central government direction, and is seemingly less able to 'think the unthinkable' at the local level. Perhaps local government has become the victim of a perverse type of 'learnt behaviour'; unwilling to be more radical at a local level since such actions are unrewarded. And, even within a post-1997 climate in which central government proclaims to take a more hands-off, facilitative and enabling approach to local action, the reality of performance management rather belies this. Certainly, the most serious obstacle to a renaissance in local government's role in local health policy is the dissonance between the 'logic' and priorities of the performance management framework and the opportunities and potential provided by democratic renewal and community governance.

NOTES

1. For more information on the history of local government involvement in health services, particularly in the inter-war period, see Webster, 1988; Eckstein, 1959; Wilson, 1946; Abel-Smith, 1964. For discussion of local government health services in the 1930s see Snape, 1995, which includes detailed case studies of health services provided by Cheshire County Council and Birkenhead County Borough.
2. It is important to state that the literature review primarily gathered evidence on the English developments, although much of the analysis is still relevant to developments in other parts of the United Kingdom.
3. Certain core Modernisation initiatives are not incorporated in this assessment – including developments in local government finance, reformed electoral arrangements and new ethical arrangements – since developments in these areas are less relevant to local government's role in health.

REFERENCES

Abel-Smith, B., 1964, *The Hospitals 1800–1948* (London).
Acheson, D., 1998, *Independent Inquiry into Inequalities in Health* (London: Stationery Office).
Armitage, L., C. Birt, H. Davis and P. Smith, 1998, 'Future Prospects for Public Health: Local Authority and Health Authority Collaboration', School of Public Policy, Occasional Paper 14, (Birmingham: School of Public Policy, University of Birmingham).
Audit Commission, 2001, *A Health Outlook: Local Authority Overview and Scrutiny of Health* (London: Audit Commission).
Audit Commission, 2002, *Comprehensive Performance Assessment: Scores and Analysis of Performance for Single Tier and County Councils in England* (London: Audit Commission).
Audit Commission, 2003a, *Patterns for Improvement: Learning from Comprehensive Performance Assessment to Achieve Better Public Services* (London: Audit Commission).
Audit Commission, 2003b, *Community Leadership*, Learning from Comprehensive Performance Assessment: Briefing 1 (London: Audit Commission).
Black, D., J. Morris, C. Smith and P. Townsend, 1980, *Inequalities in Health: Report of a Research Working Group* (London: Department of Health & Social Security).
Brown, L., C. Tucker and T. Domokos, 2003, 'Evaluating the Impact of Integrated Health and Social Care Teams on Older People Living in the Community', *Health and Social Care in the Community*, 11/2, pp.85–94.
Campbell, F. (ed.), 2000, *Building Healthy Communities: The Role of Local Government in Health Improvement* (London: LGIU).
Campbell, F., 2001, *Health and the New Political Structures in Local Government* (London: LGIU).
Carruthers, I., J. Shapter and T. Knight, 1999, *Improving Health Improvement Programmes: The Early Lessons*, Research Report 35 (Birmingham: School of Public Policy, University of Birmingham).

Clarke, M. and J. Stewart, 1998, *Community Governance, Community Leadership and the New Local Government* (York: York Publishing Services for Joseph Rowntree Foundation).
Clarke, M. and J. Stewart, 2000, 'Community Leadership', *Local Governance*, Special Issue on Local Government Modernisation, 26/3, pp.127–33.
Cramp, L., 2002, *Changing Partners: Local Government and Health in the 21st Century* (London: HDA and IDeA).
Dahlgren, G. and M. Whitehead, 1991, *Policies and Strategies to Promote Social Equity in Health* (Stockholm: Institute of Future Studies).
Department of Health (DoH), 1997, *The New NHS: Modern, Dependable*, Cm 3807 (London: Stationery Office).
DoH, 1998a, *Partnership in Action* (London: The Stationery Office).
DoH, 1998b, *Our Healthier Nation* (London: The Stationery Office).
DoH, 1998c, *Modernising Social Services: Promoting Independence, Improving Protection & Raising Standards*, Cm 4169 (London: Stationery Office).
DoH, 1999, *Saving Lives: Our Healthier Nation* (London: The Stationery Office).
DoH, 2000, *The NHS Plan: A Plan for Investment. A Plan for Reform*, Cm 4818-1 (London: Stationery Office).
Department of Environment, Transport and the Regions (DETR), 1998a, *Modern Local Government: In Touch with the People*, Cm 4014 (London: The Stationery Office).
DETR, 1998b, *Modernising Local Government: Local Democracy and Community Leadership* (London: The Stationery Office).
DETR, 2000, *Preparing Community Strategies: Government Guidance to Local Authorities* (London: DETR).
DETR, 2001a, *Local Strategic Partnerships* (London: DETR).
DETR, 2001b, *Power to Promote or Improve Economic, Social or Environmental Well-Being* (London: DETR).
Department of Transport, Local Government and the Regions (DTLR), 2001, *Strong Local Leadership – Quality Public Services*, CM5237 (London: The Stationery Office).
DTLR, 2001a, *Local Public Service Agreements: New Challenges* (London: DTLR).
Eckstein, H., 1959, *The English Health Service* (London).
Hamer, L. 2003, *Local Government Scrutiny of Health: Using the New Power to Tackle Health Inequalities* (London: HDA).
Hamer, L. and N. Easton, 2002, *Community Strategies and Health Improvement: A Review of Policy and Practice* (London: HDA/LGA/DTLR/IDeA).
Hamer, L. and J. Smithies, 2002, *Planning Across the Local Strategic Partnership (LSP): Case Studies of Integrating Community Strategies and Health Improvement* (London: HDA/DTLR/DoH/LGA/IDeA).
Health Development Agency (HDA), with the Local Government Chronicle and Health Services, 2003, *Reducing Health Inequalities: Local Government and the NHS Working Together* (London: LGC/HSJ/HDA).
Holland, W.W. and S. Stewart, 1998, *Public Health: The Vision and Challenge* (London: Nuffield Trust).
House of Commons Health Select Committee, 2001, 2nd report, January.
Hunter, D.J., 1999, 'Public Health Policies', in S. Griffiths and D.J. Hunter (eds.), *Perspectives in Public Health* (Oxford: Radcliffe Medical Press).
Hunter, D.J., 2000, 'The NHS Plan: A New Direction for English Public Health?', *Critical Public Health*, 11/1, pp.75–81.
Hudson, B., H. Lewis, E. Waddington and G. Wistow, 1998, *The Interface between Social Care and Primary Health Care: National Mapping Exercise* (Leeds: Nuffield Institute for Health, University of Leeds).
Hudson, B. and H. Lewis, 1999, *Delivering on Partnership: Social Services and Primary Care Groups* (Leeds: Nuffield Institute for Health, University of Leeds).
Hudson, B., 2002, 'Interprofessionality in Health and Social Care: The Achilles' Heel of Partnership?', *Journal of Interprofessional Care*, 16/1, pp.7–17.
Hudson, B. and M. Henwood, 2002, 'The NHS and Social Care: The Final Countdown?', *Policy & Politics*, 30/2, pp.153–66.

Hudson, B. and G. Herbert, 2003, 'Another Fine Mess', *Health Service Journal*, 30 Jan., pp.24–5.
INLOGOV, 2000, *Effective Local Strategies to Tackle the Wider Causes of Ill-Health: Research Paper* (Birmingham: INLOGOV).
Joint Review Team, 2002, *Tracking the Changes in Social Services in England*, Joint Review Team Sixth Annual Report 2001/02, Social Services Inspectorate & Audit Commission (London: Audit Commission).
Leach, S., 2002, 'Is there a Future for Overview and Scrutiny?', *Local Governance*, 28/2, pp.83–9.
Local Government Association (LGA), 1998, *A Picture of Health? A Study of Regeneration and Health* (London: LGA).
LGA, 2000a, *Partnerships with Health: A Survey of Local Authorities*, Research Briefing No 2 (London: LGA).
LGA, 2000b, *Scrutiny and the New NHS: A Joint LGA/NHS Confederation Discussion Paper* (London: LGA)
LGA, 2002, *Delivering Improvement: Local Public Service Agreements* (London: LGA).
LGA, 2002, *We Can Work it Out: In-depth Research into Development and Policy Issues for Local Strategic Partnerships*, A Report by INLOGOV (London: LGA).
Neighbourhood Renewal Unit, 2002, *Places, People, Prospects: Neighbourhood Renewal Unit – Annual Review 2001/02* (London: ODPM).
Newman, I. and M. Geddes, 2001, *Developing Local Strategies for Social Inclusion*, Local Authorities and Social Exclusion Network, Research Paper 7 (London: LGIU).
NHS Confederation (with LGA and Faculty of Public Health Medicine), 2003, *Prevention is Better than Cure: A Report from a Conference on Joined-up Thinking on Public Health* (London: NHS Confederation).
Office for Deputy Prime Minister (ODPM), 2002, *Accreditation of Local Strategic Partnerships 2001/02: An Analysis and Review of Documentation*, Research Report No. 4, Prepared by INLOGOV for the Neighbourhood Renewal Unit (London: ODPM).
Russell, H., 2001, *Local Strategic Partnerships: Lessons from the Experience of the New Commitment to Regeneration* (Bristol: The Policy Press for the Joseph Rowntree Foundation).
Snape, S., 1995, 'The Implementation of Social Policy in England in the 1930s: A Case Study of Cheshire County Council and Birkenhead County Borough' (Ph.D. thesis, University of Bristol).
Snape, S., 2000, 'Three Years On: Reviewing Local Government Modernisation', *Local Governance*, Special Issue on Local Government Modernisation, 26/3, pp.119–26.
Snape, S., 2002, 'The 14 Steps to Scrutiny Success', *Local Governance*, 28/2, pp.91–101.
Snape, S. and F. Taylor, 2001, *A Hard Nut to Crack: Making Overview and Scrutiny Work*, LGA Designing Issues in Modernisation Series (London: LGA).
Social Exclusion Unit, 2001, *A New Commitment to Neighbourhood Renewal: National Strategy Action Plan* (London: Cabinet Office).
Social Services Inspectorate, 2002a, *Modern Social Services: A Commitment to Reform*, 11th Annual Report of the Chief Inspector of Social Services 2001–2002 (London: Social Services Inspectorate).
Social Services Inspectorate, 2002b, *Modernising Services to Transform Care: Inspection of How Councils are Managing the Modernisation Agenda in Social Care* (London: DH Publications).
SOLACE, 2001, *Healthy Living: The Role of Modern Local Authorities in Creating Healthy Communities*, Report from the SOLACE Health Panel (London: SOLACE).
Webster, C., 1988, *The Health Services since the War, Volume I: The Problems of Health Care, The National Health Service before 1957* (London).
Wilson, N., 1946, *Municipal Health Services* (London).

The Health Action Zone Initiative: Lessons from Plymouth

MICHAEL COLE

The Labour government has established a wide-ranging reform agenda for the public sector (see, Cole, 2000; Cole, 2001a; Cole, 2001b; and Cole, 2002). This article considers two key aspects of this agenda through an evaluation of Plymouth's Health Action Zone (HAZ). This study concentrates, therefore, on the government's concern with evidence-based policy (Newman, 2001: 69–72) and the renewed focus on area-based partnerships as a mechanism to deliver public services (Davies, 2001).

The analysis employs a theory-based approach to evaluate the impact of a wide range of projects sponsored by Plymouth HAZ and to identify explanations. This research was generated during a three-year collaboration between the University of Plymouth and Plymouth HAZ. This article is divided into nine main sections. In the first the HAZ initiative is discussed. Section two provides information about Plymouth HAZ. Sections three and four discuss the role of HAZs as learning initiatives and the evaluation programme within Plymouth HAZ. The methodology and nature of the Plymouth study are outlined in section five. Results from the study are appraised in the next three sections. In section nine conclusions are drawn.

THE HEALTH ACTION ZONE (HAZ) INITIATIVE

The establishment of Health Action Zones (HAZs) was part of the Labour government's public sector reform agenda (Painter and Clarence, 2001). The key tenets of the modernisation thesis were outlined in a range of policy documents and White Papers (see, for example, DETR, 1998; and DTLR, 2001). In the health field this agenda included a renewed focus on health promotion and the recognition that new approaches and mechanisms might be required to tackle health inequalities and entrenched health problems in socially deprived and excluded communities.

HAZs were envisaged as a catalyst and mechanism to improve the delivery of health services. HAZs would provide a framework within which the NHS, local government and a wide range of local stakeholders could combine to address health issues. Health was, therefore, linked to employment, regeneration, education, social services, housing and anti-poverty initiatives. This agenda was part of central government's wider commitment to the delivery of public services through partnerships (Sullivan and Skelcher, 2002; and Cole and Fenwick, 2003).

This agenda also represented a commitment to area-based initiatives (DOH, 1997a; 2000). HAZs were one of several area-based initiatives (ABIs) introduced into localities with high levels of social and economic deprivation. HAZs had two strategic objectives:

> Identifying and addressing the public health needs of the local area, in particular trailblazing new ways of tackling health inequalities; and Modernising services by increasing their effectiveness, efficiency and responsiveness.

The HAZ approach was underpinned by seven principles (achieving equity; engaging communities; working in partnership; engaging frontline staff; adopting an evidence-based approach; developing a person-centred approach to service delivery; and taking a whole systems approach), which ministers asked all HAZs to reflect in their activities and plans.

Twenty-six zones were established in areas of deprivation and high health need covering over 13 million people. Fifteen HAZs were established as part of the first wave in 1998. In 1999, the Department of Health launched another 11 HAZs and ten associated HAZs, which were based in the South East region and differed from mainstream HAZs because they did not manage large funding streams.

To allow this agenda to make a significant impact, HAZs were intended to run for between five and seven years. The replacement of Frank Dobson (Secretary of State for Health 1997–99) with Alan Milburn (Secretary of State for Health 1999–2003) led, however, to a shift of emphasis within the NHS away from the broader agenda integral to HAZs in favour of a greater focus on more narrowly defined health and illness targets. The original assumption that HAZs would have a high profile in government health policy has not been reflected in the subsequent national agenda. For example, in the NHS plan, published in July 2000, reference to the specific role of HAZs was restricted to one paragraph (DoH, 2000: para.13.24).

The HAZ initiative also attracted academic scepticism. It was suggested that this agenda risked replicating the weaknesses of previous area-based/partnership-based initiatives. As Paton (1999: 65) observed, 'a reading of the history of similar initiatives does not suggest a reason for immediate optimism'. In particular, there was criticism that the projects sponsored through such structures 'created a flurry of activity, at low cost, but had little lasting impact' (Higgins, 1998: 25). In addition, it was suggested that the inter-agency tensions that characterised the earlier area-based initiatives would characterise HAZs and undermine their effectiveness. Although it was 'relatively easy to mount a collaborative bid over a short period of time ... Sustaining that level of enthusiasm and commitment over five to seven years is altogether different' (Higgins, 1998: 25).

PLYMOUTH HAZ

The award of HAZ status reflected, in part at least, local deprivation. Plymouth was one of the most deprived local authorities in England and Wales, ranking 338th out of 366 on the government's Index of Conditions. St Peter's ward was classified as the most deprived ward in England and Wales. In seven of the city's wards more than 25 per cent of households were living in poverty (Plymouth HAZ, 1998: 7).

Plymouth HAZ was established in 1998, as part of the first wave of the initiative, and had three strategic objectives:

> Developing partnership working;
> Modernising the care system; and
> Tackling health inequalities.

There were 12 programme boards. Five boards (Children and Young People; Older People; Improving Mental Health; Tackling the Problems of Substance Misuse; and Improving the Health of People with a Learning Disability) were linked to a specific user group. Another board (Oral Health) concerned a service relevant to the whole community. Five boards (Community and Voluntary Sector Development; Social Exclusion; Environment and Health; Evaluation and Research; and Improving Primary Care) had an over-arching or strategic remit. One board (Our City's Health) concerned the development of a framework incorporating 'a set of agreed targets and priorities for action to improve health and well-being and tackle inequalities' (Plymouth HAZ, 2002: 5). These boards reflected the local priority areas.

Plymouth HAZ had funded or at least attached its logo to 60 to 70 projects.[1] The list incorporated existing projects that had acquired the HAZ badge and new projects started by one of the programme boards. Each board was governed through a diverse membership reflecting the wide range of local partners. In particular, Plymouth HAZ had 'a formal policy of community or voluntary sector representation on all programme boards' (Asthana et al.: 792). The administration of the boards was conducted primarily through a Lead, invariably an employee of one of the main partners. Governance of the whole HAZ was initially through a Steering Group comprising representatives from a wide range of partner organisations. In 2000 the Steering Group was replaced by the Programme

Board Chairs' Group, which comprised the HAZ Team Leader and the chairs of each programme board. Day to day decisions were taken through the Joint Chairs' Group which comprised three individuals representing the health service, the local authority and the voluntary/community sector. The HAZ Team Leader attended these meetings.

HAZs AND EVALUATION

HAZs were conceived as learning initiatives (DOH 1997a; 1997b). Evaluation had a crucial role in the creation of this evidence base. The National Evaluation Team for the HAZ initiative selected a model for evaluation based on a combination of 'theories of change' and 'realistic evaluation' (Judge, 2000). Theories of change concerned the links between the activities, outcomes and contexts of the initiative(s) (Connell and Kubisch, 1998). In producing the theory, 'steps are taken to explicitly link the original problem or context in which the programme began with activities planned to address the problem and the medium and longer-term intended outcomes' (Judge and Bauld, 2001: 24). Theories of change concerned, therefore, how and why an initiative works (Weiss, 1995).

This approach has much in common with realistic evaluation, another theory-based framework, which tries to develop an understanding about why a programme works, for whom and in what circumstances (Pawson and Tilley, 1997). This can be summarised as the formula: Context + Mechanism = Outcome. Programmes create the mechanism and the outcome is contingent on the context. Theories of change provided the added ingredient that 'theory generation is conducted by and with those involved in planning and implementing an initiative' (Judge and Bauld, 2001: 24).

The challenge for HAZs was to articulate 'a logical way of achieving social change' (Judge and Bauld, 2001: 28) and to specify targets for each of their interventions that were stated in advance of the anticipated consequence and that formed 'part of a logical pathway that leads towards strategic goals or outcomes' (Judge and Bauld, 2001: 29).

EVALUATION AND PLYMOUTH HAZ

In Plymouth the importance of evaluation was recognised in key documents (see, for example, Plymouth HAZ, 2001: 5). The Research and Evaluation Programme Board was, therefore, well funded in comparison with the other boards. This board financed the *Learning Communities Programme* to support evaluation within Plymouth HAZ. This programme used the combined evaluation model endorsed at national level.

At first Plymouth HAZ adopted a broadly formative approach to evaluation (Bate and Robert, 2003), which was based on the notion of empowering projects to evaluate their interventions. An Evaluation Adviser was appointed to facilitate this process and the projects asked to conceptualise their interventions in terms of theories of change and realistic evaluation. In particular, each project was sent a monitoring and evaluation form, which requested basic information and was constructed in terms of the theory-based model.

Unfortunately, most projects were reluctant to engage with this process. A key problem was the failure of over three-quarters of the projects to return the monitoring and evaluation form.[2] A decision by the Programme Board Chairs' Group that projects were required to return the form was, therefore, not implemented. This initiative was undermined by several factors. First, the Evaluation and Research Programme Board failed to promote the importance of evaluation within Plymouth HAZ. Many participants regarded evaluation as irrelevant. A key player in the evaluation process commented that many people at the operational level resented the amount of money allocated to evaluation and that 'there was a feeling within HAZ that it is about delivering services and that money not spent on delivering services is, therefore, not spent in the right way'.

Second, *Learning Communities* was undermined by the 'changing composition of the board and the absence of a dedicated lead' (Cole, 2003a: 14). Third, most practitioners were unable to handle the theory-based approach. For example, a senior manager in a statutory agency observed that his/her board members had struggled to understand a presentation about theories of change and the evaluation strategy (Cole, 2003a: 14). Fourth, there was a mismatch between the agenda of *Learning Communities* and the work of the other agencies. Staff typically gave evaluation a low priority because it was viewed by most senior managers as either irrelevant or a threat. Fifth, in attempting to impose a common framework for evaluation, *Learning Communities* was insensitive to the diversity of projects. In particular, expecting recipients of very small grants to engage with this approach could be criticised as unrealistic.

After almost two and a half years of the three-year programme, *Learning Communities* had generated almost no information about the success or failure of Plymouth HAZ's projects.[3] Specific projects and boards had conducted evaluations separate from *Learning Communities*. These initiatives were, typically, inadequate. Most were superficial and insufficiently critical. None employed a theory-based approach.

THE STUDY AND METHODOLOGY

This study is the result of the third stage of *Learning Communities,* which involved an evaluation of the projects sponsored by five programme boards (Improving Primary Care; Oral Health; Children and Young People; Older People; and Substance Misuse). These boards were selected to reflect the range of work undertaken by Plymouth HAZ. The research incorporated 37 HAZ projects. The analysis used the list supplied by the HAZ Team (Plymouth HAZ, 2002). Two of these projects were, however, omitted from the study. Both the *Over 75 Survey* and *Tackling Isolation* were excluded because they were not specific HAZ projects but pieces of work that had been 'spun off' existing projects. The study did, however, incorporate three projects that were not identified by the HAZ Team.[4]

The analysis was based primarily on semi-structured interviews with key participants. Interviews were held with 72 individuals between 19 September 2002 and 27 February 2003. The interviews ranged in length from 15 minutes to almost two hours. Initial interviews were held with the Lead of each board to obtain a comprehensive list of projects funded by each board, initial indications about achievements and problems and the name of one individual or, at least, organisation responsible for each project. Where it was not possible to speak to an individual with responsibility for the project a person with substantial knowledge was substituted. This approach retained the theories of change/realistic evaluation model; however, it was primarily non-interventionist and retrospective. This evaluation incorporated characteristics of both summative and formative approaches (Bate and Robert, 2003).

The interviews with these *project people* focused on the achievements of each project, the problems encountered, the impact and the extent of user involvement. The first *project person* interviewed about a specific project was asked for the name(s) of other individual(s) who could speak about the initiative. This 'snowballing' approach was crucial in securing an adequate list of interviewees. This strategy also enabled the study to obtain a more detached and objective perspective and balance the tendency of those responsible for projects to emphasise achievements to the exclusion of problems. However, although a few *project people* were defensive and reluctant to discuss problems, in general the interviews were characterised by transparency and openness. The selection of interviewees also reflected the requirement to obtain the views of people from a wide range of different organisations. In particular, the representation of employees from the statutory health sector was restricted to under half the sample, while almost of a third of these participants worked for community or voluntary organisations (see Table 1). This work was supplemented with a wide range

TABLE 1
HAZ INTERVIEWEES BY SECTOR OF EMPLOYMENT

Sector	Interviewees
Statutory Health	34
Statutory Social Services	7
Statutory Education	3
Statutory Other	1
Community/Voluntary	22
Private Sector	5
Total	72

of documentation about specific projects (see, for example, Plymouth HAZ, 1998; Plymouth HAZ, 2001; Garlick, 2001; and Borbon, 2002). This article also incorporates evidence from the strategic evaluation (Cole, 2003a).

The projects were evaluated in the context of three themes. First, the documentation and interviews were assessed to identify the presence of a theory of change/realistic evaluation approach. Second, projects were evaluated in terms of the extent to which they achieved their aims and the extent to which these initiatives contributed towards the three key objectives of developing partnership working, modernising the care system and tackling health inequalities. Third, reasons for the success or failure of projects were identified.

A THEORY OF CHANGE AND REALISTIC EVALUATION APPROACH

Despite the failure of most projects to complete the evaluation and monitoring form or identify the context, mechanism or outcome, the documentation showed that in many projects significant links had been made between activities/mechanisms, outcomes and contexts (see Connell and Kubish, 1998). Some projects drew on theories of change models taken from national government. For example, the Smoking Cessation project drew on a theory of change and evidence-based model of guidance that the Department of Health had instructed HAZs to follow when establishing local services (Raw et al., 1998; and Judge and Bauld, 2001). Similarly, the initiative to integrate equipment services drew on Department of Health guidelines, which incorporated a theory of change (DOH, 2001).

The Integrated Substance Misuse Service project also developed a theory of change/realistic evaluation framework with distinctive context, mechanism and expected outcome elements (S&WDHA, 2000). However, the implementation of this agenda suffered because the initial plan was too simplistic. It comprised targets and deadlines but lacked a detailed framework about how to achieve them. The participants underestimated the problems of attempting something that had never been attempted before in the UK – 'the creation of an integrated substance misuse service in the voluntary sector' (Cole, 2003b: 101).

The interviews showed that most projects had been justified in terms of an approach that could be structured into a context/mechanism/outcome model. For example, the establishment of a vocational dental training scheme was set in the local context of an ageing population of dentists in Plymouth, the absence of a training scheme based in the city, the difficulty of attracting qualified dentists to the city, the need to strengthen or at least maintain the level of NHS dentistry in the city and substantial inequalities in the local provision of oral health care. The mechanism was identified as the establishment of the vocational training scheme and outcomes were provided in the form of the number of trainees that decided to remain in the city after qualification and the impact on the provision of NHS dentistry in Plymouth.

A context, mechanism and outcome framework was also present in the development of the work programme of the HAZ boards. For example, the programme of the Substance Misuse Board was placed in the context of high drug use in Plymouth. Mechanisms to address the problems were identified in the form of interventions such as the establishment of an integrated substance misuse service, the creation of community-focused networks to support substance misusers, the development of a co-ordinating structure across all specialist services, and the development of 'a robust system for user and carer involvement in service development decisions' (Plymouth HAZ, 1998: 40). In addition, outcomes were specified. Targets included reducing referrals to substance misuse services and increasing the proportion of schools 'with appropriate programmes of drug education in place' (Plymouth HAZ, 1998: 41).

ACHIEVEMENTS

The 36 projects that had been substantially completed were evaluated in terms of the extent to which they had achieved their objectives. Projects were classified through the use of six categories (see Table 2). The analysis showed that 28 (78 per cent) of the projects had achieved substantial success in meeting their objectives. Several HAZ sponsored projects had a significant impact on an issue important to the health and social care community. Prominent examples included RITA and the Integrated Substance Misuse Service.

Plymouth Rapid Response (RITA)

The project prevented many inappropriate admissions of older people to Derriford hospital.[5] The project involved the establishment of a multi-

TABLE 2
ACHIEVEMENTS

Degree of Success	Projects
Yes (S)	10
Yes (ST)	11
Yes (S?)	2
Yes (NS)	5
Mod (Led)	2
Little	6
Total	36

Notes:

Yes (S) = Achieved substantial success in meeting its objectives and was sustained by an agency(ies).

Yes (ST) = Achieved substantial success in meeting its objectives and was conceived as a primarily short-term initiative.

Yes (S?) = Achieved substantial success in meeting its objectives. Sustainability is possible but not confirmed.

Yes (NS) = Achieved substantial success in meeting its objectives but was not sustained.

Mod (Led) = Achieved modest success in meeting its objectives but contributed towards successful developments in the field.

Little = Achieved little success in meeting its objectives.

disciplinary team of health and social care professionals. The team investigated and arranged alternatives to admission to Derriford for older patients referred from GPs. This strategy involved the establishment of the first GP-controlled beds in a Plymouth hospital and the funding of alternative care packages. This success was recognised in 2001 when the scheme was the runner-up in the NHS South West Modernisation Awards.

Integrated Substance Misuse Service

The initiative involved the establishment of an integrated service that incorporated voluntary and statutory agencies. The integration process overcame a history of mistrust and antagonism between the component agencies and drew on the expertise of a wide range of professionals. Integration highlighted important problems that had been obscured, identified solutions and improved the accessibility of the service. For example, the changes 'led to information sharing, the identification of waiting times as a significant problem and showed that this latter difficulty could not be resolved without changing working patterns' (Cole, 2003b: 99).

However, only ten (28 per cent) of these projects were evaluated as having been sustained by an agency after the HAZ funding expired. Eleven projects (31 per cent) were conceived primarily as short-term initiatives. Examples included the Baseline Epidemiology project, which involved a survey of the oral health of five year olds in the city, the Minor Injuries Unit – Children's Video project, which involved the dissemination of information about the Minor Injuries Unit to children and the production of a video, and the scoping study consultation on fluoridation, which consisted of a survey of the attitudes of the key agencies towards fluoridation of Plymouth's water supply.

Another five (14 per cent) of these successful projects were envisaged as long-term initiatives but failed to secure long-term funding from the key agencies. Important examples included the Parenting project and Resources for Health Workers in the Community.

Parenting Project

This initiative focused on the development of 'consistent and quality services to support parents' (Plymouth HAZ, 2002: 60) and aimed to make Plymouth a 'parent-friendly' city. Key outputs included 12 basic principles or quality standards, known as the Plymouth Principles, and a directory of parenting organisations. Parents were incorporated into the decision-making process and substantial work was undertaken on establishing a Parenting Forum for the city. However, the Forum was never established because the project ended when the HAZ finance expired. The end was accompanied by acrimony. The project's steering group was very critical of key agencies and suggested that HAZ funding had been wasted. In particular, the parent participants, most of whom represented the socially excluded and deprived communities prioritised by HAZ, 'ended the process cynical and disillusioned' (Cole, 2003b: 74). In contrast, the agencies emphasised the refusal of the project manager to try to raise funds from other sources and the constraints on their budgets.

Resources for Health Workers in the Community

This project enabled community health care workers to place children in a nursery in response to health needs. Before the HAZ initiative access had been restricted to social care requirements and directed through Social Services. The objective of the HAZ finance, which ceased after six months, was to highlight the value of the service and persuade the local Primary Care Group to provide all the funds. However, the Primary Care Group was 'unable to give guaranteed long-term funding only six monthly extensions after often intensive lobbying from individuals involved with the project' (Cole, 2003b: 42). The process of acquiring funds was a drain on the project and was resented by key personnel. One interviewee observed that, although she recognised the value of the scheme, she would have refused the HAZ finance if she had realised the effort required to sustain the initiative. In late 2002 the Primary Care Group announced that funding would cease.

Two projects (six per cent) achieved only modest success in meeting their objectives but could be viewed as making a significant contribution to a wider agenda. For example, the immediate impact of the Hepatitis C Development project, which sought to explore the impact of a positive Hepatitis C diagnosis on clients participating in drug treatment, was reduced by problems with the methodology of the research and the reluctance of drug workers to attend the training. It was, however, plausibly argued that the project helped to push Hepatitis C up the local policy agenda and contributed to the decision to appoint a dedicated Hepatitis C worker in Plymouth, the only such appointment south and west of Bristol.

Six projects (17 per cent) achieved little success in meeting their objectives. Examples included Offbase, which aimed to establish information about the requirements of young people who used drugs, alcohol and other substances. The two partner agencies lacked 'any common concept' (Cole, 2003b: 107) about the project, the project team strayed beyond their remit and the initiative collapsed without achieving important objectives. Similarly, an attempt to establish a drug Service Users' Action Group generated a small and ineffective group that collapsed within a few months.

The projects were also evaluated in terms of their contribution to the three strategic objectives of Plymouth HAZ: developing partnership working; modernising the care system; and tackling health inequalities.

Developing Partnership Working

Plymouth HAZ made an important contribution towards developing effective partnership working in the city. HAZ acted as a catalyst for the partnership approach to public service provision and served as the mechanism to bring together individuals who should have been working in partnership. Plymouth's approach acquired a national reputation and was praised by a government facilitator as 'more sophisticated than in other HAZs' (Cole, 2003b: 11).

Partnership working fostered an enhanced sense of trust among the participants. One key player in Plymouth HAZ commented that there was 'a lot of trust around' (Cole, 2003b: 11). A colleague observed that they had 'now reached the stage where we can openly criticise what perhaps other agencies are doing without taking it personally' (Cole, 2003b: 11).

The partnership agenda also strengthened the position of users and carers within the decision-making process. This change improved the governance of health and social care because users and carers typically brought a different perspective to the decision-making process. In addition, participation at this level enabled users and carers to appreciate the constraints under which the professionals worked and promoted mutual trust between the two 'sides' (Cole, 2003b: 11).

Positive partnership working has been expressed through a wide range of projects. Examples included the service integrations and other multi-agency initiatives such as RITA. In addition, many projects were facilitated through multi-agency steering groups and collaborations between professionals. Examples included Resources for Health Workers in the Community, the Parenting project and the Integrated Substance Misuse Service.

Modernising the Care System

Plymouth HAZ had a significant impact on modernisation of the health and social care system. HAZ sponsored projects made important contributions to piloting and the development of service integration in areas such as substance misuse and children's services. For example, it was suggested that without HAZ it would have been impossible to have established an integrated substance misuse service because there would have been insufficient trust amongst the relevant agencies. HAZ improved the lines of communication between them, 'dealt with suspicion, dealt with competition with a small 'c' and tried to develop a holistic view ... on how is the best way to deal with drug and substance misuse' (Cole, 2003b: 10).

Other projects modernised services through increasing co-operation and co-ordination between different agencies/disciplines. For example, RITA modernised the delivery of services relevant to a client base of elderly and vulnerable people, while the Primary Care Assessment Link Workers Scheme concerned the development of new models of working that improved the delivery of services through enhanced liaison between GPs and Social Services. HAZ projects also modernised the delivery of services in isolation, examples included the development of a Smoking Cessation team and the establishment of a family therapy service in primary care.

HAZ provided the catalyst to introduce modernisations to tackle problems that had been recognised but unresolved for many years. For example, HAZ provided the catalyst to tackle problems around the use and management of equipment. The intervention of HAZ also led to the establishment of a successful project about the handling of asthma issues in schools. In contrast, a similar project ten years before had achieved little.

Tackling Health Inequalities

The evaluation produced evidence that some HAZ projects had generated outcomes relevant to the health inequalities agenda. For example, NHS dentistry, which had a disproportionate client base among deprived and socially excluded individuals, was enhanced through the establishment of a Dental Access Centre and a vocational dental training scheme (Cole, 2003b). The Welfare Benefits Sustainable Take-Up Campaign raised benefit take-up among elderly people in Plymouth. Similarly, the Child Wise Parenting project improved the parenting skills of some of the most socially excluded and deprived people in the city.

The impact of HAZ sponsored projects was, however, affected by a range of factors. First, tackling health inequalities is a long-term process and benefits of HAZ projects, in general, could not be quantified until the projects and, probably, HAZ had ended. Second, in many cases the impact of a specific HAZ initiative on health inequalities was difficult or impossible to quantify. Third, there was evidence of imprecision in the way some projects approached the issue.

These problems can be illustrated through an analysis of Grab Five, which aimed to increase the consumption of fruit and vegetables amongst primary school-aged children. Although there is a consensus that increasing the consumption of fruit and vegetables by children will have health benefits, accurate quantification of the effect is impossible. First, to assess the impact these children (or a sample) would have to be monitored for decades. Second, isolating the impact of the HAZ would be impossible. Third, although the project was targeted on schools in deprived areas some incorporated catchment areas with a significant minority of children from more affluent backgrounds.

These difficulties had a marked impact on the manner in which Plymouth HAZ addressed this objective. First, there was a notable tendency amongst some partners to link any quantifiable reduction in health inequalities in a relevant area with a HAZ initiative. Second, there was an emphasis on arguing that activities of the projects represented a direct contribution to tackling health inequalities. For example, in the absence of statistics for the relevant period, the development of innovative mechanisms to communicate with young people about contraception was seen as a direct contribution to reducing health inequalities in this area. Third, there was also an emphasis on tackling health inequalities through taking the initial step of acquiring baseline information. Fourth, some participants argued that closing gaps in service provision through initiatives such as the Asthma Schools project, which focused on improving service provision for children with asthma, contributed to tackling health inequalities regardless of the impact on different socio-economic groups.

The analysis produced some evidence of a direct and quantifiable impact on health inequalities, however; in general, it was not possible to quantify the impact of HAZ initiatives. Evidence for the impact of HAZ on health inequalities in Plymouth was typically indirect and concerned with interventions rather than measurable reductions.

EXPLAINING SUCCESSES AND FAILURES

The study identified a range of explanations for the success or failure of projects.

National Policy Agenda

The success of some of the most important projects was linked to a specific national initiative. The renewed national focus on the development of NHS dentistry was identified as a key factor in the establishment of a Dental Access Centre at Mould Gould. Similarly, Grab Five benefited from an emphasis on promoting healthy eating amongst children adopted by the Department of Health. The Smoking Cessation project was part of an independent national scheme that was assigned to the city because Plymouth had a HAZ and an Education Action Zone (EAZ).

National Service Frameworks also motivated some projects. For example, a project that focused on reducing admissions to hospital among people over 60 years reflected, in part at least, the National Service Framework for the Care of Older People (Cole, 2003b: 81–4).

Local Policy Agenda

The analysis showed that the local policy agenda had positive and negative effects on projects. For example, the Citywide Bed Management project, which concerned the implementation of a co-ordinated plan for the management of health and social care beds in Plymouth, was, in part at least, a response to a crucial problem for the key agencies. Similarly, the Welfare Benefits – Sustainable Take-Up Campaign benefited from the legacy of a previous initiative (PWRSU, 2000). In contrast, the low priority given to parenting issues explained the failure of the key statutory agencies to finance the Parenting project after the HAZ funding ended.

Trust

The success of multi-agency projects was facilitated through the development of trust amongst the partners. Overcoming a tradition of mistrust among the relevant agencies was the essential prerequisite for the establishment of the Integrated Substance Misuse Service. Similarly, the development of trust was crucial to the Citywide Bed Management project because the process through which teams at Mount Gould and Derriford hospitals acquired an understanding of the problems facing each other involved the development of a substantial degree of trust between them. The lessons from Plymouth HAZ confirmed, therefore, the academic literature about the importance of trust to public sector management (Coulson, 1998).

Cultural Convergence

Multi-agency projects often required the partners to overcome cultural and linguistic difficulties. The success of collaborations between health and social care professionals were typically dependent on overcoming significant difficulties. In particular, it was essential to reconcile social and medical models of care and persuade participants that they had to modify their working methods to accommodate people from different disciplines. Such co-operation can lead to the establishment of new and integrated models of working which combine the strengths of each partner. For example, the creation of the Integrated Substance Misuse Service drew on the relative equality in the relationship between clients and professionals in the voluntary sector and the clinical expertise of the statutory health care professionals.

Cultural convergence often involved changes to the role(s) performed by professionals. For example, cultural convergence between statutory and voluntary sectors through the establishment of the Integrated Substance Misuse Service led health professionals to accept that non-nurses could manage nurses.

Expertise

The skills of key personnel were a crucial determinant of success. In particular, research-based projects often suffered from the weak research skills of health and social care professionals with responsibility for the work. This issue reflected wider weaknesses in the research capacity of many public sector organisations (Sanderson *et al.*, 2001; and Cole, forthcoming).

The appointment of non-specialists could, however, lead to innovation and improved methods of working. For example, the non-NHS or local authority background of the project manager was cited as a reason for the success of the Citywide Bed Management project. He approached issues free of the preconceptions held by most health and social care professionals.

Managerial Clout

The presence of advocates in senior management can be crucial to the success of projects. The Treatment of Mild to Moderate Depression project, which aimed to improve treatment through counselling, benefited from the strong support of a senior NHS manager and suffered when that individual departed to another job. In contrast, the junior status of one project manager meant that (s)he had little credibility with senior management in the local authority or hospital consultants.

Engagement with Crucial Agencies and or Individuals

The success of most projects was dependent on engaging a wider group of individuals/organisations and placing health issues onto the agenda of other agencies. For examples, Grab Five and the Baseline Epidemiology Study depended on the participation of schools. This requirement meant that most projects had to develop effective mechanisms to engage with those participants. Many projects had to acquire sensitivity to the time constraints of the partner organisations/individuals and their often marginal stake in, or enthusiasm for, the relevant project. In particular, questionnaires had to eschew jargon and be as succinct as possible. Long and technical questionnaires typically produced low response rates and generated unreliable data.

The analysis revealed several examples of how problems with access to external agencies/groups reduced the impact of projects. For example, the impact of the Oral Health Workplaces project, which took the oral health message to workplaces in the city, was limited substantially because the team was unable to access an appropriate list of contacts and some participating workplaces refused to engage with the evaluation (Cole, 2003b: 58–9). Community Solutions to Teenage Pregnancy encountered problems in engaging with 'young people in a meaningful manner' (Cole, 2003b: 16). Similarly, the credibility of the drug Service Users' Action Group was undermined by the failure of the activists to engage with the wider community of users.

Managerial Structure

Clear responsibilities, line management and accountability were prerequisites for a successful project. Absence of such structures typically caused difficulties. For example, the problems experienced by Offbase were linked to a flawed managerial structure that was 'an inelegant compromise without any common concept about the service to be delivered' (Cole, 2003b: 107).

Legal Constraints

A court case led to the suspension of the 'Morning After Pill' project, which concerned the availability of contraception, while copyright problems delayed the production of the Oral Health Information Folder. Similarly, the refusal of the Department of Health to grant a dispensation to allow the Integrated Substance Misuse Service to be established in the voluntary sector delayed the creation of the service.

CONCLUSIONS

The results from Plymouth illustrate the potential and limitations of area-based initiatives to deliver improvements in public services. In general, the study suggests that the traditional scepticism of the academic literature may need to be modified. In particular, such wide-ranging partnerships appear to be useful as a catalyst to promote joint working between agencies. The analysis showed that partnership at board level promoted the development of a co-operative culture that assisted the establishment of integrated services and the other multi-agency projects. There was also evidence that Plymouth HAZ helped to shift some local policy agendas and assisted in the resolution of long-standing problems.

The analysis has also generated important conclusions about the role of evidence in the development of policy and the influence of other factors. While there was evidence of processes and reasoning that can be linked to a theory of change/realistic evaluation framework, enthusiasm for rigorous evaluation was limited. A wide range of factors affected the impact of projects. For example, many of the most successful projects benefited from a strong national agenda. Similarly, success was also affected substantially by the wider agenda of the key local agencies. In particular, the long-term impact of HAZ was reduced by the refusal of the main agencies to sustain some successful initiatives after the HAZ funding ended. The analysis also identified the difficulty of using a short-term initiative such as HAZ to tackle problems such as health inequalities, which are the consequence of a wide range of social, economic and cultural influences and are difficult to influence within a short timeframe.

NOTES

1. For example, three projects in this evaluation received no finance from HAZ.
2. Most of the returned forms were not completed adequately.
3. *Learning Communities* was structured into three stages. The first stage (May 2000 to October 2001) focused on facilitating the evaluation process and developing capacity. The second stage (October 2001 to July 2002) concerned a strategic evaluation. In the third stage (July 2002 to April 2003) 37 HAZ projects were evaluated.
4. Grab Five; the Dental Access Centre; and the Detox Support and Relapse Prevention project.
5. Derriford is the main hospital in Plymouth.

REFERENCES

Asthana, S., S. Richardson and J. Halliday, 2002, 'Partnership Working in Public Policy Provision: A Framework for Evaluation', *Social Policy and Administration*, 36/7, pp.780–95.
Bate, P. and G. Robert, 2003, 'Where Next for Policy Evaluation? Insights from Researching National Health Service Modernisation', *Policy and Politics*, 31/2, pp.249–62.

Borbon, J., 2002, *The Impact of a Hepatitis C Diagnosis on Treatment for Substance Use* (Plymouth: The Eddystone Trust).

Cole, M.S., 2000, 'The Cole Report: Report on the Role of Members and the Modernising Agenda', unpublished report commissioned by Devon County Council.

Cole, M.S., 2001a, 'Executive and Scrutiny Reforms: The Agenda and its Impact at Devon County Council', *Local Government Studies*, 27/4, pp.19–34.

Cole, M.S., 2001b, 'Local Governmental Modernisation: The Executive and Scrutiny Model', *The Political Quarterly*, 72/2, pp.239–45.

Cole, M.S., 2002, 'The Relationship between County Councillors and Other Tiers of Elected Local Government; The Case of Devon', *Local Governance*, 28/2, pp.103–13.

Cole, M.S., 2003a, *Learning Communities Report – HAZ: A Strategic Evaluation* (Plymouth: Department of Sociology, University of Plymouth).

Cole, M.S., 2003b, *Learning Communities Report – HAZ: A Project Evaluation* (Plymouth: Department of Sociology, University of Plymouth).

Cole, M.S., 'Consultation in Local Government: A Case Study of Practice at Devon County Council, *Local Government Studies* (forthcoming).

Cole, M.S. and J. Fenwick, 2003, 'UK Local Government: The Impact of Modernization on Departmentalism', *The International Review of the Administrative Sciences*, 69/2, pp.259–70.

Connell, J.P. and A.C. Kubisch, 1998, 'Applying a Theory of Change Approach to the Evaluation of Comprehensive Community Initiatives: Progress, Prospects, and Problems', in K. Fulbright-Anderson, A.C. Kubisch and J.P. Connell (eds.), *New Approaches to Evaluating Community Initiatives: Volume 2, Theory, Measurement and Analysis* (Washington DC: The Aspen Institute).

Coulson, A. (ed.), 1998, *Trust and Contracts: Relationships in Local Government, Health and Public Services* (Bristol: The Policy Press).

Davies, J.S., 2001, *Partnerships and Regimes* (Aldershot: Ashgate).

Department of the Environment, Transport and the Regions (DETR), 1998, *Modern Local Government: In Touch with the People*, Cm 4014 (London: HMSO).

Department of Health (DOH), 1997a, *The New NHS: Modern, Dependable*, Cm 3807 (London, The Stationery Office).

Department of Health (DOH), 1997b, *Health Action Zones – Invitation to Bid*, EL(97)65, 30 October (Leeds: Department of Health).

Department of Health (DOH), 2000, *The NHS Plan: A Plan for Investment, A Plan for Reform*, Cm 4818-1 (London: The Stationery Office).

Department of Health (DOH), 2001, *Guide to Integrating Community Equipment Services* (London: Department of Health).

Department for Transport, Local Government and the Regions (DTLR), 2001, *Strong Local Leadership – Quality Public Services*, Cm 5327 (Norwich: The Stationery Office).

Garlick, S., 2001, *Consultation on Water Fluoridation* (Kingsteignton: Hygiene 2 Health).

Higgins, J., 1998, 'HAZs Warning: The White Paper Debate', *Health Service Journal*, 16 April, pp.24–5.

Judge, K., 2000, 'Testing the Limits of Evaluation: Health Action Zones in England', *Journal of Health Services Research and Policy*, 5/1.

Judge, K. and L. Bauld, 2001, 'Strong Theory, Flexible Methods: Evaluating Complex Community-Based Initiatives', *Critical Public Health*, 11/1. pp.19–38.

Newman, J., 2001, *Modernising Governance: New Labour, Policy and Society* (London: Sage).

Painter, C. and E. Clarence, 2001, 'UK Local Action Zones and Changing Urban Governance', *Urban Studies*, 38/8, pp.1215–32.

Paton, C., 1999, 'New Labour's Health Policy: The New Healthcare State', in M. Powell (ed.), *New Labour, New Welfare State?* (Bristol: The Policy Press), pp.51–75.

Pawson, R. and N. Tilley, 1997, *Realistic Evaluation* (London: Sage).

Plymouth Health Action Zone, 1998, *Plymouth Health Action Zone Implementation Plan, January 1999 to April 2000* (Plymouth: Plymouth Health Action Zone).

Plymouth Health Action Zone, 2001, *Plymouth Health Action Zone: Programme Board Pack*, 1st Edition (Plymouth: Plymouth Health Zone).

Plymouth Health Action Zone, 2002, *HAZ Project File* (Plymouth: Plymouth Health Action Zone).

Plymouth Welfare Rights Support Unit (PWRSU), 2000, *Over 60s Benefit Campaign* (Plymouth: Plymouth Welfare Rights Support Unit).

Raw, M., A. McNeill and R. West, 1998, 'Smoking Cessation Guidelines for Health Professionals: A Guide to Effective Smoking Cessation Interventions for the Health Care System', *Thorax*, 53/1, pp.S1–S9.

Sanderson, I., J. Percy-Smith and L. Dowson, 2001, 'The Role of Research in "Modern" Local Government", *Local Government Studies*, 27/3, pp.59–78.

Sullivan, H. and C. Skelcher, 2002, *Working Across Boundaries: Collaboration in Public Services* (London: Palgrave).

South and West Devon Health Authority (S&WDHA), 2000, *Report on Creation of a Single Substance Misuse Agency in the City of Plymouth, South Hams and West Devon* (Plymouth: South and West Devon Health Authority).

Weiss, C.H., 1995, 'Nothing as Practical as Good Theory: Exploring Theory-Based Evaluation for Comprehensive Community Inititatives for Children and Families', in J.P. Connell, A.C. Kubisch, L.B. Schorr and C.H. Weiss (eds.), *New Approaches to Evaluating Community Initiatives: Concepts, Methods and Contexts* (Washington DC: The Aspen Institute).

Overcoming the Desire for Misunderstanding through Dialogue

PAUL HOGGETT

EXTERNAL CONSTRAINTS ON PARTNERSHIP

No one needs reminding how much talk there is these days about the need to 'think outside your boxes', engage in 'joined up' thinking and action, get beyond a 'silo mentality' and so on. Of course nothing is new about this; policy-makers complained about the scourge of departmentalism back in the 1970s when Corporate Management was seen as the answer to the problem of co-ordination and integration in government (Clapham, 1985). What is striking, then, is just how obdurate this problem has been, how remarkably resilient to transformation the systems of governance appear to be. Why is this?

One line of analysis looks at actors in terms of interests and motives. Here our attention is directed to issues such as the way in which different parts of government, such as health and local government, while being exhorted to work together effectively are also having to dance to quite different tunes being played by Whitehall pipers who are far from being in tune themselves. In other words, because they have very different agendas imposed on them, different priorities, different timescales, and so on, there are real material constraints upon their capacity to work in concert. Coming down a level, the NHS and local government constitute different administrative cultures, with different languages and ways of seeing the world. Again this provides a material basis for misunderstanding, as often occurs, for example, when different actors operate with quite different notions of 'accountability', one thinking managerially, the other thinking in terms of representational politics. We might also think in terms of the existence of 'structural interest groups' (Alford, 1975; Friedson, 1994; North and Peckham, 2001) such as the professions engaged in competitive struggle for territory or in terms of the different 'domains' (Kouzes and Mico, 1979) – policy, service and so on – that make up systems of public governance. Finally, at the micro-level of specific institutions in particular localities, these will have their own internal institutional politics, power struggles and 'ways of doing things' which are uniquely theirs. In other words, at macro-, meso- and micro-levels there are plenty of material factors which make inter-organisational co-operation difficult. There is nothing new about this, it has always existed. The problem is, knowing that it exists does not really help local actors who wish to or need to co-operate.

THE MYTH OF THE INCLUSIVE COMMUNITY

There has to be a desire for change. This is easily said. What does it mean? It means that there has to be a desire to embark upon a course of action in full knowledge of the difficulty and of the risks that will be incurred. It is easy to talk glibly about change, perhaps particularly when Blairites are inclined to talk blithely about 'embracing change', as if change was simply a matter of seizing opportunities which had not been grasped largely because of our own inadequacy. This kind of triumphalism does not help. It does not help because it seems blind to what we might think of as the 'dark side' of change – the precariousness of it, the risks that actors are exposed to and not just from the 'other side' but from 'their own camp'. But then this is a government which is pretty uncomfortable with conflict. I am thinking here specifically of a kind of deep-seated communitarianism which imagines a political community, both nationally and locally, in essentially consensual ways. Let me pause just for a moment. Since the seminal work of Benedict Anderson it has become accepted by most social theorists that all communities, from the nation state to the village, are first and foremost imagined communities (Anderson, 1983). Labour, then, tends to imagine communities as places where everyone can belong, and where the interests of some do not pose a fundamental constraint upon the inclusion of others: as if there are no real material conflicts of interest, for example, between the needs of an increasingly globalised capital and the needs of the socially excluded or, at a local level, as if communities themselves were not riddled with competing interests and incommensurable identities and ways of living. The point is that social change, that is, change in the patterns of social relatedness in which we are all caught up, is an essentially conflictual process. And the problem is that conflict rests very uneasily within Labour's political philosophy. Indeed, the very modernisation of Labour, the transformation of its own internal processes of governance, has been designed to avoid open conflict within the party itself (Webb, 2000).

This has major implications for the way in which Labour construes public participation and social inclusion. Indeed, Labour is the first British government to frame public participation explicitly in terms of social inclusion (Levitas, 1998). In other words, participation is framed consensually as a way of drawing the excluded and disaffected into an imaginary common community. This article offers a quite different perspective, one that sees conflict as an inherent aspect of all social relations. Indeed, this article will argue that conflict is something which is necessary for the creation of real and enduring forms of social solidarity (Simmel, 1955) – between communities and between actors in different organisations. Without the conflictual negotiation and renegotiation of relationships, social bonds become superficial, more simulated than real, indeed sometimes a mask which conceals ongoing processes of disintegration.

COMMUNITY WITHOUT UNITY

There is a huge public housing estate in South Bristol which has been riven by generational conflicts for some time. To the adult residents it seems like some groups of young people are out of control. Public space, particularly at night, is seen as unsafe; vehicles are regarded as fair game to be driven away by young men and trashed; open spaces, schools, youth clubs and community centres are subject to constant vandalism, and so on. But when youth workers tried to intervene by getting tough with the children they found that local adults would often quickly take the side of the young people, a solidarity forming almost instantly against the professional 'outsiders'. Clearly the conflict between generations is partly built upon real differences of interest. Young people feel that there is nothing for them to do, no one is interested in them or understands them, people simply want to 'slag us off'; adults feel that their property is insecure, women and older people in particular feel that the area has been made unsafe.

But it is the ease with which these conflicts of material interest are abandoned in favour of a common unity of 'locals' against the outsider which perplexes youth and community workers (and local teachers) and makes their job all the more difficult. And this takes us to a quite different level of analysis, to processes of identification and the complex mixture of permanence and fluidity that characterise them – in this case, to the enduring identity of the 'local', something built upon shared class and life experience, whose power is momentarily able to transcend generational forms of difference.

Generational conflicts dominate the estate but they are by no means the only kind. Differences are felt according to which part of the estate you live in, main roads becoming important territorial markers whose significance is entirely lost to the outsider; differences are felt according to cultural background – refugees and asylum seekers, particularly from a Muslim background, becoming the new 'blacks' on the estate;[1] and then, of course, there are the traditional differences built upon gender, with strong, female-dominated, extended kinship networks constituting the backbone of social welfare on the estate (Gill, 2000). Closer to the ground there are clear distinctions made between 'rough' and 'respectable' families, and then there are some 'notorious' families who are linked to organised crime. This estate is no different to many other largely white, working class estates in Bristol, such as the Southmead estate in the north of the city. Speaking of Southmead, Jeremy Brent uses the phrase 'community without unity' (1997). In sharp contrast to communitarian ways of thinking Brent argues that 'exclusion and splitting, rather than union, is constitutive of community' (p.73). It is worth stopping to think about this. In contrast to current policy-think, which sees inclusion and harmony as constitutive of community Brent is arguing the opposite, that community exists (as a shared sentiment and construct) because of (not in spite of) exclusion and splitting.

SPLITTING AND EXCLUSION IN THE WELFARE PROFESSIONS

It is possible to take this idea a bit further and apply it not just to local residential communities but to local occupational communities such as those to be found gathering behind organisational boundaries which mark off the health service from local government, health visitors from general practitioners, youth workers from teachers, and so on. To understand why 'joined up' thinking and action between different professional groups is so difficult, to understand why it inevitably involves conflict, we need to think about it differently and we need to draw upon perspectives which are themselves different to those that we are used to (for example, the sociology of community, the psycho-dynamics of inter-group behaviour, theories of identity and difference).

So, in what ways are imagined local occupational communities brought into existence and sustained by virtue of processes of exclusion and splitting? This question will be explored by using another case study, this time of the interaction between a community mental health team and an in-patient ward team which covered the same sector of a city (Daum, 2002). In reality, there was an enormous inter-dependence between these two teams, not the least because when patients were discharged from the ward they became the responsibility of the community team and, vice versa, when the community team could no longer contain patients in their care these patients were typically hospitalised. However, actual relations between the two teams were marked by hostility, misunderstanding and non-cooperation. What was at work here? Daum worked with each team in order to understand what he called their 'relationship-in-the-mind', that is, the experience, partly conscious and partly unconscious, they had of relating to the other team. Daum points out that the predominantly female ward team performed their task in an old psychiatric institution hidden away in the country, three miles out from the city boundary and safely split off from the consciousness of its inhabitants. They had to work with adults in their most regressed and dependent state in contrast to the community team (the majority of whom were male) whose task was to support patients in their efforts to live independently in the community. All psychiatric nurses, as part of their career progression, had to 'cut their teeth' on the ward and as a result many community staff felt that they were 'one up from' but had also 'escaped from' the ward. Ward staff were seen as less professional and this was mirrored in complaints about their disorganisation. Working with inquiry groups involving members of both teams and making use of visual imagery as well as verbal methods of eliciting data, a number of powerful images were generated of this 'relationship-in-the-mind'. One of them was particularly vivid, namely

> a shared fantasy amongst community staff that ward staff spend their time in the office drinking cups of tea and smoking cigarettes, whilst ward staff harbour the conviction that community work allows staff to have lengthy, undisrupted meetings away from patients ... before going out to lunch in a nice trendy cafe that truly bears no resemblance to the hospital canteen. (Daum, 2002)

Daum uncovered a dynamic of envy and resentment between the two teams which often became manifest in rivalry for the attentions of the consultant psychiatrist to whom both teams were responsible.

If we look at processes of identity formation and maintenance within this occupational community, Daum suggests that the community team managed to sustain a collective belief in their own professional competence by splitting off their sense of failure and impotence (a result of the chronic and enduring nature of the emotional difficulties facing many of the patients, which, combined with the inadequate resourcing of community care, produced a high re-admission rate) and locating it in the ward team who consequently could do no right. In contrast, the ward team were stuck in and with madness on a daily basis. Its largely female staff were consigned to largely physical and technical caring tasks with frightened and frightening adults and came face-to-face with the sometimes traumatic aspects of psychiatry – compulsory admission, the administration of ECT, the unmistakeable impacts of strong doses of psychotropic drugs and so on. In the face of such unbearably bad experiences the ward team struggled to maintain some sense of coherence and morale – a struggle greatly facilitated by the proximity of the arrogant, uncomprehending community team which becomes construed in a wholly persecutory way. By locating many of their bad feelings in the community team, the ward staff are able to avoid enough of the bad feelings generated by the job to be able to cope. By getting rid of and splitting off certain feelings and locating them in the other team, each team can generate a sense of 'we-ness'. In other words, onto the actual differences of each team (differences located in the role they perform, the occupational skills and experience they draw upon, and so on) are loaded a set of imaginary differences and it is in the latter, not the former, where problems of misunderstanding become generated. In order to preserve its own identity each group tacitly manifests a desire to misunderstand the other.

CONFLICTUAL DIALOGUE

Although some readers may feel that this is a very particular kind of example, such processes of splitting and projection occur all the time between groups and communities which share the same social space. Freud once called it 'the narcissism of minor differences'. Some people are inclined to call such phenomena dysfunctional. Such rationalist and consensualist perspectives fail to appreciate the satisfactions to be derived from splitting and exclusion. We enjoy our petty dislikes and intense hatreds. As in the example above, these processes are often very functional for the part, though unfortunately not for the whole. The problem is that in most organisational and inter-organisational spaces these imaginary differences go unacknowledged, participants having little reflexive awareness of the dynamics that are at work. Moreover, there is a fear that open communication about such things, which will inevitably have a conflictual dimension to it, will lead to irreparable damage. Again, such fears drive actors towards a rationalist position which says if only people would leave their emotions out of this and we all focused upon the practical task at hand then everything would be okay. To hear managers say this kind of thing (as they often do) is reminiscent of the celebrated librarian who insisted her library would be fine if people did not keep coming in to use the books, or, in other words, organisations would function fine if they were not filled with human beings. So instead of a conflictual dialogue between groups what tends to emerge is a kind of lifeless consultation, strong on form (after all there are so many techniques available for consulting these days) but weak on substance; one which gives people the feeling of being included (Chandler, 2001) but denies the groups concerned the enormously important experience of having a conflict, surviving it and growing from it. Before developing this point it is important to examine how groups and individuals learn from experience.

There are two kinds of learning – learning about the other and learning from the other. Conventional social sciences such as policy studies and organisational studies can tell us a great deal about the other. Such forms of 'objective knowledge' as those listed at the beginning of this article provide us, for example, with an understanding of some of the constraints which act against more integrated forms of policy action and programme delivery. But such forms of knowledge do not in and of themselves lead to change in our pattern of social relatedness because they provide understanding about external constraints rather than internal resistances. If a group is to change the way in which it relates to other groups then it must also learn from the other. An organisation may know a great deal about its service users without learning from its users – if it is to learn from experience then it must find ways of integrating 'learning about' and 'learning from' – that is, objective knowledge and subjective knowing. The crucial difference between the two kinds of learning is that learning about the other does not necessarily entail learning about self, whereas learning from the other necessarily entails learning about self. This is why it is more difficult. Wherein does the difficulty lie?

If 'we' are to learn from 'them' then we must be capable of having an encounter with a 'them' which is something more than a bundle of our projections; in other words we must be capable of engaging in a real dialogue with a real 'other' rather than an imaginary dialogue with an imaginary 'other'. Groups do this all the time – engage in imaginary dialogues. We can catch ourselves doing this when, in fantasy, we conduct a conversation with members of another organisation which is a potential partner or rival. In the conversation, the participants in the dialogue take up certain positions, this is what Daum means by the 'relationship-in-the-mind'. In the case of the teams in his study, members of the ward team engaged in imaginary relations with an arrogant and uncomprehending community team, whereas members of the community team engaged with an inadequate and over-dependent ward team. The identity of each team leant upon the way it construed the other. So there was a collusion going on; neither team felt understood by the other and perversely this suited them all (only the organisation as a whole and the users of its service suffered). For a change in the pattern of relatedness to occur, each team not only had to be prepared to have its perception of the other challenged, each team also had to undergo a challenge to its own self-perception, that is, to its own identity.[2] Learning from the other therefore presents a double challenge, and if change is to occur it requires a conflictual renegotiation of ways of seeing both other and self (Maoz et al., 2002). This is the real meaning of dialogue, and it is difficult precisely because of the anxieties it evokes. As the misunderstandings generated by group identities are tackled, the foundation is laid for open negotiation around conflicts of material interest.

Because of the anxiety it evokes, many communities, including occupational communities, prefer to fight or engage in relations of mutual misunderstanding rather than engage in conflictual dialogue. And knowing about the fear that fuels hostility, resentment and non-cooperation enables us to be clearer about some of the conditions necessary for change to occur. If groups are to become more aware (in today's jargon we would say 'become more reflexive') about themselves and their way of relating to others they must have some way of containing this anxiety. Some groups have a developed internal capacity for doubt and openness to new experience, but where this is absent or weakly formed or where the stakes involved in the inter-group encounter are high then this capacity will to some extent have to come from outside. Considerable thought therefore needs to be given to the creation of an environment in which the anxieties provoked by conflictual dialogue can be contained.[3] There are many practical steps to consider here, including the way in which inter-group meetings are structured and chaired, the ground-rules that need to be accepted as appropriate rules of conduct by the parties concerned, the use of external facilitation, and so on. Many of these ideas are familiar to those engaged in conflict management and the mediation movement and many find expression in the practices of some of the newer social movements (Schlosberg, 1995).

OCCUPATIONAL BOUNDARIES AND PARTNERSHIP WORKING

This article deliberately draws attention to some of the difficulties of working across boundaries that are often overlooked. By examining the way in which community boundaries are developed and sustained we are more able to appreciate the role of inter-group dynamics in reinforcing fragmentation and non-holistic forms of working. In a recent review of the history and present state of partnership working, Hudson and Henwood (2002) indicate how some of the real material constraints upon partnership between health and social care have been tackled by recent government legislation which has, for example, facilitated funding transfers between the NHS and local government. However, the authors also note recent signs of a return to some very old solutions, and specifically the idea that restructuring and reorganisation can finally bring about more holistic approaches. The resort to this kind of structural solution must prompt feelings of despair in anyone who has been around long enough to observe the failure of previous such strategies. Drawing on the experience of Northern Ireland, where Health and Social Services Boards have operated for many years, Hudson and Henwood (2002) note that 'structural integration evidently does not guarantee co-ordinated practice on the ground'. Drawing on Clarke and Stewart's work on 'wicked issues', they note that the key challenges facing partnership working today are precisely the 'soft' issues explored in this article – differences in perspective between different occupational communities; tolerating, not knowing and accepting differences; inclusivity as opposed to exclusivity; and the ambivalence actors feel when faced with the challenge of real learning as opposed to what we might think of as 'going through the motions of learning'. In the light of these challenges, Hudson and Henwood conclude that 'organisational structures and boundaries (and any reshuffling of them) becomes a secondary matter'.

In conclusion, let us return to the nature and dynamic of conflicts between communities in residential areas. Bauman (1995) talks about the fear and hostility generated by the stranger who does not fit in with us and the desire to obliterate this difference either by assimilation or by expulsion. Although the stakes are not so high, one can see similar processes at work in encounters between different occupational groups, particularly the belief that if only we could make 'them' more like 'us' then collaboration could occur. Respecting the other's difference, welcoming the opportunity to work with difference and being able to tolerate the discomfort and uncertainty it will bring does not come easily. If we accept that all identities are to some extent built upon processes of exclusion and splitting, then to learn from another who is different means taking back into ourselves things that we find difficult to bear. It means abandoning some of the comforting illusions that 'our group' holds about itself. It means re-taking ownership of that which we have disowned and placed in the other 'so that the stranger outside is no longer identical with the strange within us' (Benjamin, 1998: 108).

NOTES

1. I use 'black' here as a racialised category that can be inhabited by a variety of ethnic minority groups according to which at a given time and in a given place is the primary target for inferiorisation and hatred (see Jeffers *et al.*, 1996).
2. Elsewhere I have suggested that this imagined identity assumes the form of an 'internal establishment' which can impose a kind of tyrannical 'group think' upon group members. See my chapter 'The Internal Establishment' in Hoggett, 2000.
3. By 'contained' I do not mean 'suppressed'; the notion of 'containment' comes from psychoanalysis where it refers to the human capacity to provide safe, resilient and flexible support. See Hoggett and Thompson (2002) for a discussion of the role of containment in facilitating deliberative democracy.

REFERENCES

Alford, D., 1975, *Health Care Politics: Ideological and Interest Group Barriers to Reform* (Chicago: University of Chicago Press).

Anderson, B., 1983, *Imagined Communities: Reflections on the Origins and Spread of Nationalism* (London: Verso).

Bauman, Z., 1995, *Life in Fragments* (Oxford: Blackwell).

Benjamin, J., 1998, *The Shadow of the Other* (New York: Routledge).

Brent, J., 1997, 'Community Without Unity', in P. Hoggett (ed.), *Contested Communities* (Bristol: Policy Press).

Chandler, D., 2001, 'Active Citizens and the Therapeutic State', *Policy and Politics*, 29/1, pp.4–14.

Clapham, D., 1985, 'Management of the Local State: The Example of Corporate Planning', *Critical Social Policy*, p.14.

Clarke, M. and J. Stewart, 1997, *Handling the Wicked Issues: A Challenge for Government* (Birmingham: University of Birmingham).

Daum, M., 2002, 'Dangerous Liaisons: Projective Identification, Envy, and the Conflict between Love and Hate in the Relationship between Two Psychiatric Teams', *Organisational and Social Dynamics*, 2/1, pp.120–38.

Friedson, E., 1994, *Professionalism Reborn: Theory, Prophecy and Policy* (Cambridge: Polity Press).

Gill, O., C. Tanner and L. Bland, 2000, *Family Support: Strengths and Pressures in a 'High Risk' Neighbourhood* (Ilford, Essex: Barnardos).

Hoggett, P., 2000, *Emotional Life and the Politics of Welfare* (Basingstoke: Macmillan).

Hoggett, P. and S. Thompson, 2002, 'Towards a Democracy of the Emotions', *Constellations*, 9/1, pp.106–26.

Hudson, B. and M. Henwood, 2002, 'The NHS and Social Care: The Final Countdown', *Policy and Politics*, 30/12, pp.153–66.

Jeffers, S., P. Hoggett and L. Harrison, 1996, 'Race, Ethnicity and Community in Three Localities', *New Community*, 22/1, pp.111–26.

Kouzes, J. and P. Mico, 1979, 'Domain Theory: An Introduction to Organisational Behaviour in Human Service Organisations', *Journal of Applied Behavioural Science*, 15/4.

Levitas, R., 1998, *The Inclusive Society? Social Exclusion and New Labour* (London: Macmillan).

Maoz, I., S. Steinberg, D. Bar-On and M. Fakhereldeen, 2002, 'The Dialogue between the 'Self' and the 'Other': A Process Analysis of Palestinian–Jewish Encounters in Israel', *Human Relations*, 55/8, pp.931–62.

North, N. and S. Peckham, 2001, 'Analysing Structural Interests in Primary Care Groups', *Social Policy and Administration*, 34/4, pp.426–40.

Schlosberg, D., 1995, 'Communicative Action in Practice: Intersubjectivity and New Social Movements', *Political Studies*, 43, pp.291–311.

Simmel, G., 1955, *Conflict and the Web of Group-Affiliations*, Tr. from German by R. Bendix (London: Collier-Macmillan).

Webb, P., 2000, *The Modern British Party System* (London: Sage).

Leading and Managing at the Boundary: Perspectives Created by Joined Up Working

MIKE BROUSSINE

In their candid moments, chief executives will testify to their role being both the best and also the hardest in local government. They will admit to contrasting experiences in occupying the role. These represent in themselves emotional 'boundaries', like having power to influence things and make things happen *and yet* also feeling powerless sometimes; identifying considerable achievements which contribute to the local authority's effectiveness, *and yet* feeling that they are often in a 'no-win situation'.

This article resulted from being asked by the Society of Local Authority Chief Executives (SOLACE) to facilitate reflection on the changing role of the local authority chief executive. It therefore concentrates on this role. However, anecdotal evidence suggests that chief and senior executives in other agencies face similar dilemmas.

The reflections in this article have not been formed through a single piece of systematic research. The ideas arise from numerous interactions with chief executives and directors in various settings – in one-to-one supervision sessions, informal talks, critical reflection in learning sets, and the comments of some chief executives and SOLACE members on earlier drafts of this article. Thus the methodology may be seen as a form of *action inquiry* (Torbert, 1991; Reason, 1998) in which the data is generated 'on-line' through a lived experience – in this case of regular and frequent interaction with local authority chief executives over the past four years. Torbert argued that action inquiry differs from orthodox scientific research in that it is concerned with 'primary' data encountered through the lived experience, and only secondarily with recorded information. With regard to the reflections offered in this article, the data is related to theoretical analyses that offer insight into a complex structural, emotional, political system in which traditional boundaries are increasingly being questioned.

The article is structured as follows: a brief overview of what is meant by joined up working is presented; the dual nature of the chief executive's role is considered; an analysis of the chief executive's boundary role provoked by joined up government is provided; three particular aspects of this boundary role are explored in depth – buffering and boundary spanning, knowing and not knowing and leading and managing; and the article concludes by examining the practical implications for the role and development of chief executives.

JOINED-UP-NESS AND THE LOCAL AUTHORITY CHIEF EXECUTIVE

Organisation theory has recognised in recent years that the traditional boundaries of organisations have become increasingly complex:

> as organisations form strategic alliances ..., erasing boundaries which separated them, or alternatively setting up internal markets and agencies which erect new internal boundaries ... the idea that an organization is separated from its environment by a fixed line has become increasingly unhelpful under such conditions. (Gabriel, 1999: 97)

Inherent in the notion of 'joined up' government are the concepts of:

* multi-agency working
* 'seamless' delivery
* governance
* democratic renewal
* community leadership
* permeable organisational boundaries
* partnership

> A local authority partnership is a process in which a local authority works together with partners to achieve better outcomes for the local community, as measured by the needs of the local stakeholders, and involves bringing together or making better use of resources. This working together requires the development of a commitment to a shared agenda, effective leadership, a respect for the needs of the partners, and a plan for the contributions and benefits of all the partners. (DETR, 1999: 5)

The concept of 'joined up' government holds the prospect of increased complexity in chief executives' and senior managers' role. In a workshop at the SOLACE Conference in Newport in September 1999, partnership, multi-agency working, joined up or seamless government suggested a system of 'unimaginable complexity' to Simon White, Director of Social Services at the London Borough of Camden. First, he suggested that there were several types of joined up government, for example, pooled budgets, lead commissioning and integrated provision. Second, cultural differences between partnership organisations were inevitable. His experience suggested that, generally speaking, local government tends to be vocal about duties, while health tends to be vocal about effectiveness. He argued that, while central government's rhetoric about partnership is simplistic – sometimes partnerships are not possible – the 'complexity of human need' in society was such that it had to be addressed by arrangements that transcend organisational boundaries.

'Joined-up-ness' suggests that, somehow, numerous public, private and voluntary systems and sub-systems may be meshed together in a series of complex relationships in order to impact beneficially on society and the citizen. Many of the chief executives the author has talked to thought that these developments held potentially profound implications for their roles. Moreover, joined up government cannot be examined in isolation from other fundamental political and structural changes that have been introduced, especially the introduction of new democratic structures in local authorities. These changes, taken together, will make special demands on chief executives' roles. They are already leading to fundamental questions about the nature and purpose of the chief executive's position. The questions that were raised by a sample of leading elected members during earlier research for SOLACE (Broussine, 2000) – 'Do we need a chief executive or a different animal?' and 'Will they [chief executives] be required in the future?' – seem relevant now.

DUALITY IN THE ROLE OF CHIEF EXECUTIVE

Effective joined up working rests to some extent on the personal authority of the chief executive – that is, on her or his ability to represent or embody the interests of the entire organisation. The capacity 'to develop effective external relationships' was one of the five key capacities uncovered in the earlier research for SOLACE (Broussine, 2000). That capacity included a number of descriptors which included 'Being a champion of the local authority, local government and local democracy' and 'Working with communities and other agencies'.

The conclusion of this earlier research was that the complex and dynamic role of a chief executive needs to be seen in its totality, as a *Gestalt*. Therefore, it was inappropriate to see chief executives' capacities in isolated ways: 'the capacities and their associated capabilities inter-relate and manifest themselves in an almost limitless fashion' (Broussine, 2000: 507). If we concentrate on the capacity to work with other agencies as an important corollary of 'joined up government', there are (at least) two kinds of leadership required:

- one which concerns itself with community and governance – leadership in relation to the *external* world;
- another which is concerned with the *internal* structure and culture of the local authority itself.

It is this duality of role that contributes to the complex and paradoxical nature of the chief executive's job. To put it in the most basic terms, a local authority cannot work effectively with its external world unless it has its internal act together (a point to which the article returns later). The chief executive therefore occupies a role at the boundary of the internal and external worlds of the organisation. This is also true for chief officers and directors who, similarly, occupy particular spaces in both of these worlds. It may also be true to an increasing extent for those local political leaders who hold positions as executive members in cabinets, and it is important to realise that this particular aspect of role is not confined to the chief executive alone. However, there are special demands made of the chief executive who regards him or herself as working at the interstices of management and politics as part of a dynamic set of relations which incorporates both elected members and officers. The duality of role that is held by the chief executive is therefore not a constant. How and what is held or given priority will be subject to an interchange between the chief executive and the part s/he plays. Fox and Leach pointed to the difficulty in predicting the effects of changes in political structures on the chief executive's role:

> Some interviewees predicted that the new arrangements would lead to chief executives playing more of an internal co-ordination and arbitration role and spending less time outside an authority and promoting community governance. ... However ... [other] interviewees believed that the new arrangements would occupy members to such an extent in other matters that chief executives/officers will need to spend even more time brokering partnerships and networking. (Fox and Leach, 1999: 40)

THE CHIEF EXECUTIVE'S BOUNDARY ROLE

The concept of boundary implies a transitional space that contains ambiguity and 'unknowing'. A boundary shows how different worlds relate to each other. It is where representatives of different identities meet. Boundaries provide us with defences against anxiety, and yet their existence causes anxiety. We need boundaries, but they also get in the way of joined up working. They both help us to define the identity of those worlds, and to redefine their changing relationship. This is important because, as we have seen, the internal and external worlds of the local authority are shifting. Perceptions of the nature of boundaries similarly will not remain constant. A person who can work effectively at the boundary is trying continuously to make sense of what is going on there in a situation of flux.

For all these reasons, it is important that the chief executive is aware of the nature of the structural, political and psychological boundaries he or she encounters in the interacting and overlapping systems s/he works in. The demands that being at the boundary make on the chief executive can be seen, in the short run, as a clash or choice between competing priorities. In the longer term, to see the complexity of leading at the internal/external boundary as merely a choice of priorities at any moment is naive. How can a chief executive take the lead in joined up working with other agencies when her or his local authority is itself not internally joined up? In my various interactions with chief executives it seemed that a new emphasis was being placed on *corporate management* in the leadership of the local authority's internal structure and culture.

Working at the boundary suggests a need to be able to manage with the internal strengths and weaknesses of the local authority, and at the same time lead in the midst of the dynamics that inter-agency and partnership working provokes. This means being able to hold several capacities simultaneously – buffering and boundary spanning, 'knowing' and 'not knowing', and leading and managing.

Buffering and Boundary Spanning

Buffering involves protecting the internal operations of the organisation from interruption by 'environmental shocks'. *Boundary spanning* describes the activity of environmental monitoring, scanning *and* representing the organisation or its interests to the environment (Hatch, 1997). The boundary spanning role may be performed by a number of specialists employed by the local authority (depending on size) whose primary concerns are with the transfer of data and information across the organisational boundary, for example public relations officers, policy officers.

The 'protecting' role in buffering requires the capacity to absorb the complexities and ambiguities of a changing environment. While this role is actually performed by a number of people in the organisation as they carry out their operational tasks, the emotional demands that uncertainty and ambiguity make become greater for those working at the top of the organisation. Arguably buffering not only requires the capability to work with the external world of parish councils, other public, private and voluntary organisations, citizens and communities, but also to have the emotional capacity to hold competing and irreconcilable demands and pressures simultaneously.

The Boundary between 'Knowing' and 'Not Knowing'

There is much pressure on senior managers to show that they 'know' – that is, to demonstrate that they are in control of, and have knowledge about, what is going on in their internal and external domains. These pressures to show that they know can come from at least three sources:

- from within the organisation (it is unsettling for staff in a dependent and hierarchical structure to feel that their boss does not know the answer);
- from elected members (some members hold an assumption that senior managers and chief executives are – or ought to be – omniscient);
- from within the person (the need to avoid looking incompetent or foolish) – Senge (1990) discussed how, even if we feel uncertain or ignorant, we learn to protect ourselves from the pain of appearing uncertain or ignorant.

Given the nature of the local authority's external environment, senior executives cannot possibly know or predict everything – the earlier discussion about the complexities involved in working at the boundary showed why this is not possible. Nearly all chief executives recognised this; but they also recognised that they were often under considerable pressure to 'know'. The ability to sustain the pretence of knowing is, however, limited and can lead to intolerable emotional demands.

Managers' obsession to know can be regarded as a form of psychosis: a strong feeling of uncertainty or ambiguity leads to a need for more and more information. The more information and data that is gathered, the more the environment will seem complex and changing, which in turn leads to a continually expanding search for yet more data. Not only can this be a form of personal psychosis, but, if held by a chief executive or director, can transfer into a form of organisational psychosis and goal displacement as well.

Chief executives and other senior managers need to be able to see the boundary between 'knowing' and 'not knowing' as a potentially fruitful place to be (French and Simpson, 1999):

> The boundary is the best place for acquiring knowledge. ... Since thinking presupposes receptiveness to new possibilities, this position is fruitful for thought; but it is difficult and dangerous in life which again and again demands decisions and this excludes alternatives. (Paul Tillich, 1967: 13)

Paradoxically, the chief executive can, through demonstration of tolerance of 'not knowing', encourage people in the local authority and in other agencies to be receptive to new ideas, to be creative – to think. That is not to minimise the emotional and political difficulties of achieving this: as French and Simpson (1999) suggested, the key is to be aware that this boundary has the potential for both creativity and terror.

In these days of lower job security for chief executives, the state of unknowing described here could so easily be misinterpreted as incompetence or indecisiveness. Traditionally, 'knowing' has been a source of power and authority. However, working at this transitional space offers a relevant and practical kind of organisational and inter-organisational leadership which joined up government and further 'environmental shocks' require. It is a kind of leadership that is based on self-knowledge, inner confidence and a good enough sense of identity instead of pretence and obsession with getting it right and being in control all the time.

The Boundary between Leadership and Management

The third boundary chief and senior executives need to be at is that between management and leadership. As we have seen, the question of leadership is crucial when the chief executive or director is working at the boundary. Farey's (1993) analysis of the difference between leadership and management is useful to us. He ascribed the notion of 'transformational leadership' to the role and purpose of *leadership*, and 'transactional leadership' to those of *management*. Farey (1993; quoting Burns, 1978) suggests that transformational leadership involves the capacity of leaders to have their goals clearly and firmly in mind, to fashion new institutions relevant to those goals, to stand back from immediate events and day-to-day routines and understand the potential and consequences of change. By contrast, transactional leadership may be seen as fulfilling the rational managerial functions of the systematic development of strategies to achieve goals, the deployment of resources, the design, organisation, direction and control of the activities required to attain goals, and motivating and rewarding of people to do the work.

The distinction between management and leadership is now widely acknowledged and used in management education. Most chief executives the author talked to could associate themselves with the analysis. We have to be careful not to fall into the trap of seeing the leadership as residing only at the apex of the organisation, in the chief executive. However, the distinction frees us to ask questions such as whether or not organisations are over-managed and under-led (Bennis and Nanus, 1985), and whether or not the roles of leadership and management are invariably held in the same person.

The distinction between transformational and transactional leadership represents another important boundary for the chief executive. How s/he perceives the boundary is wrapped up in her or his self-identity, which will affect the style with which the role is exercised. It will affect how the task of working in partnership with other agencies is constructed in his or her mind. Is partnership working, on the one hand, seen as new, radical, risky, uncertain, creative, looking outside current parameters or constraints – in short, requiring transformational leadership? Or, on the other hand, is it seen as a means of acquiring resources, increasing efficiency, reducing costs and solving today's rather than tomorrow's problems – requiring transactional leadership? The answers to such questions have the potential to exert considerable influence on the workings of partnerships and multi-agency arrangements. Awareness of being at this, and the other boundaries, gives the chance for productive and creative thinking.

PRACTICE IMPLICATIONS FOR THE ROLES AND DEVELOPMENT OF CHIEF EXECUTIVES

Chief executives will need increasingly to have to capacities to:

- understand the permeability of the local authority's organisational boundaries – this may manifest itself in increasing ambiguity or leakage in role;
- recognise cultural differences across and between boundaries and sectors;
- pay simultaneous attention to both the internal and external worlds they work in – to focus on relations with other agencies in order to attain joined up government while ensuring that the local authority itself is internally joined up;
- have a tolerance of ambiguity and uncertainty: recognising that such complexity may be best understood by attempting not to seek resolutions to problems too hastily, but staying with the creative possibilities that awareness of being at a boundary entails;
- recognise the impossibility of omniscience – of knowing (and controlling) everything that is going on – in a complex and changing world, and developing a capacity in oneself and in others to tolerate 'not knowing' as a basis of sense-making, reflection and creativity;
- place a new emphasis on *corporate management* in the leadership of the local authority's internal structure and culture;
- buffer and boundary span – this means developing the emotional capacity and resilience to hold competing and irreconcilable demands and pressures simultaneously.
- recognise that, if the chief executive's role is about working at the structural, political and psychological boundaries of the role and of the organisation, not all the demands of domains they work with are reconcilable.

How might chief and senior executives develop the awareness necessary to achieve these capabilities? There are two connected means: to appreciate the need for systemic analysis and to maintain personal perspective, self-knowledge and sense-making. Each is considered in turn below.

Systemic Analysis

By trying to see the *Gestalt* – the connections within and between the various systems at play in and between organisations (and their sub-systems) – chief and senior executives may be able to use their experience to understand in some depth what is going on in a complex organisation with both fixed and permeable boundaries. In systemic analysis, each part of what is going on affects other things going on. The idea of inter-related parts emphasises that, while all systems can be broken down for the purposes of analysis, their essence can only be understood when the system is looked at as a whole. So the duality of the chief executive's role is itself a systemic concept.

To comprehend a system, we must transcend the view of individual parts to encounter the whole system at its own level of complexity. To understand the external environment of the local authority, we must also understand how the authority both affects, and is affected by, that environment. Hirschhorn and Gilmore (1992) argued that when work interactions go horribly wrong, people can become frustrated, angry, confused and even ashamed. But such feelings, they suggest, are not just the inevitable emotional residue of human work relationships. They are *data*, valuable clues to the dynamics of boundary relationships. So, feelings – including one's own possibly intense emotions – are an aid to thinking, managing and leading. To be a good boundary manager, they argued, executives must be able to decipher frustrating and difficult personal relationships and diagnose why they have gone wrong. The implication is that senior managers need to be able to develop the capacity to see how their own responses are symptoms of broader organisational processes. Hirschhorn and Gilmore concluded that awareness of feelings, one's own and others', is crucial to making flexible organisations work.

For example, there may be intense antipathy towards the voluntary organisation, the health service or local community groups with whom the local authority is seeking to work. What is causing these feelings? Is it because of 'personalities'? Do some random historical occurrences or relationships cause the antipathy? Or does the antipathy tell us something important about both the constraints to, and possibilities of, partnership working? Alternatively, does it tell us about the pressures potential partner organisations are experiencing? Assuming that the people involved are not incompetent or mischievous, something in the systems represented is causing these intense feelings. The ability to make sense of such questions lies at the heart of working effectively at the boundary.

Maintaining Personal Perspective and Self-Knowledge

The earlier research for SOLACE identified the capacity for maintaining personal perspective and self-knowledge as one of the five capacities which were thought central to the chief executive's effectiveness (Broussine, 2000). To repeat an earlier point, a person who can work effectively at the boundary is trying continuously to make sense of what is going on there in a situation of flux. How might the chief executive develop his or her capacity for sense-making and holding a sense of her or his identity? The earlier research indicated that the capacity for maintaining perspective was made up of 'maintaining self-knowledge', 'maintaining belief or faith in self', and 'developing personal resilience'.

The product of maintaining personal perspective may not necessarily result in immediately positive outcomes. In certain cases, the changes which are being brought about by the modernisation agenda may create a feeling of dissonance between a chief executive's self-identity and the new reality, to the extent that some may not be able to tolerate their lesser role (if that is what it is to be). Fox and Leach (1999) found there was a fear that the chief executive's role will be less prominent or important in the future, and that some may depart the job as a result. Despite (and because of) these pressures, this third capacity has become increasingly important as the local government system encounters the strategic shocks and 'unimaginable complexity' which are beginning to shake assumptions about the nature and purpose of the role.

It is therefore not surprising that increased numbers of chief executives and their colleagues are participating in development and learning strategies such as learning sets, personal role supervision and mentoring, each of which in their way provides the space for checking out self-identity, increasing self-knowledge and for reflecting critically on structural and emotional boundaries. Chief executives need increasingly to see their leadership and managerial role as one that requires self-knowledge, inner confidence and a 'good enough' sense of identity. What it comes down to is this – that effective work at the new boundaries which joined up government requires means that we have to see leadership and learning as simultaneous if not synonymous activities.

CONCLUSION

Many chief executives see the complexity of the role – in a context of joined-up-ness and working at the boundary between politics and organisational leadership – as having to work in the space between contested value judgements while simultaneously maintaining their own perspectives and holding on to faith in their own judgements. When reflecting on their roles, they will describe themselves sometimes as being the man or woman in the middle – at the boundary – between conflicting and committed views of how problems should be solved. In one learning set, chief executives discussed the notion of being 'two-faced', asking themselves how they could work with integrity between a demanding and vocal group of elected members and an anxious staff group. It would be easy to surrender one's own identity and integrity by, at different moments, appearing to side with one group or the other. In practical terms, chief executives were sensitive to the dangers of moaning about members when they were with their officer colleagues, or *vice versa*. Leading *at* the boundary – rather than avoiding it – requires the chief executive to hold on to what s/he stands for. The chief executives I have worked with all, in their different ways, have recognised the need to revisit regularly what it is that brought them into local government in the first place, and what hopes they have about the system which they have a pivotal role in leading.

REFERENCES

Bennis, W. and B. Nanus, 1985, *Leaders: The Strategies of Taking Charge* (New York: Harper & Row).
Broussine, M., 2000, 'The Capacities Needed by Local Authority Chief Executives', *International Journal of Public Sector Management*, 13/6, pp.498–507.
Burns, J.M., 1978, *Leadership* (New York: Harper & Row).
DETR, 1999, *A Working Definition of Local Authority Partnerships*, research on behalf of DETR conducted by Newchurch and Co. Ltd.
Farey, P., 1993, 'Mapping the Leader/Manager', *Management Education and Development*, 24, Part 2.
French, R. and P. Simpson, 1999, 'Our Best Work Happens When We Don't Know What We're Doing', ISPSO 1999 Symposium, 25–27 June.
Fox, P. and S. Leach, 1999, *Officers and Members in the New Democratic Structures* (London: Local Government Information Unit).
Gabriel, Y., 1999, *Organizations in Depth* (London: Sage Publications).
Hatch, M.J., 1997, *Organisation Theory – Modern, Symbolic and Postmodern Perspectives* (Oxford: Oxford University Press).
Hirschhorn, L. and T. Gilmore, 1992, 'The New Boundaries of the "Boundaryless" Company', *Harvard Business Review* (May–June), pp.104–15.
Reason, P., 1998, 'Three Approaches to Participative Inquiry', in N.K. Denzin and Y.S. Lincoln (eds.), *Strategies of Qualitative Inquiry* (London: Sage), pp.261–91.
Senge, P.M., 1990, *The Fifth Discipline: The Art and Practice of The Learning Organisation* (London: Century Books).
Tillich, P., 1967, On *the Boundary: An Autobiographical Sketch* (London: Collins).
Torbert, W.R., 1991, *The Power of Balance: Transforming Self, Society, and Scientific Inquiry* (Newbury Park, CA: Sage).

Partnerships between Health and Local Authorities: Concluding Remarks

PAT TAYLOR

As a concluding note it is useful to reiterate Lyn Harrison's summing up from the first Bristol ESRC seminar in March 2000. Lyn's comments were made on the basis of extensive involvement in evaluating and acting as a consultant to joint working over 20 years. Her remarks were enthusiastically received by the participants at the seminar who were, mainly, practitioners centrally involved in implementing the partnership agenda and they indicate well the complexity of the factors influencing partnership working

Having just undertaken a systematic review on joint working (Cameron, 2000) she injected a note of caution into the enthusiasm for joint working by pointing out that 'despite the proliferation of guidance and good practice handbooks there is in fact little evidence of the effectiveness of joint working'. Lyn commented that:

* *We need to be 'smarter' about knowing when to develop partnerships and when to find other ways to achieve identified goals.* We need to know which problems are best tackled by joint working. We also need to be clear about which level of the organisation needs to be 'joined up'. A 'jointness' may be better at a strategic level with operational levels playing to their strengths within a 'joined up' framework. It is important to assess how many collaborative ventures can be supported within any one area so that when new partnerships are required it may be essential to ask if there is an existing one that will do.

* *We need to create and reward, through training and career development, a pool of workers skilled in supporting joint working.* Currently it is usually chance that someone with the skills and understanding is available to provide facilitation and leadership in partnership working. Partnership working skills have not been necessarily part of current management or professional training. Health and local authorities have much to learn from the networking and entrepreneurial skills of private, voluntary and community organisations.

* *We need to evaluate more systematically the effectiveness of joint working.* We need to know more about the tangible short and long term

benefits for service users and communities from joint working initiatives. We need to be clearer and more honest about the real resource costs of joint working. The history of joint working indicates that short term funding initiatives will not automatically lead to changes in the core business of agencies or mainstream budgets.

- *The significance of the boundaries and differences which block joint working cannot be underestimated.* Many boundaries have been created over decades and are reworked daily through myths and stereotypes and are not going to be changed lightly. Boundaries are where power is exercised by control of budgets, professional practices, eligibility criteria and access to services. Altruism is not the dominant motivation for professionals and therefore it cannot be assumed that they will be driven to work together solely by the desire to contribute to the well being of the population. The problems, which are evident in current service provision and the difficulties which have historically existed over joint working indicate that the institutional and professional landscape is structured inappropriately. This would suggest in theory that there is a need for a dramatic reconfiguration of the main agencies commissioning and delivering services. In theory this could lead to very large benefits but in practice would be a very *high risk strategy.*

Lyn finished with three quotes which make a fitting conclusion to this volume:

Use formal partnerships selectively and review frequently. (Audit Commission, 1998)

Don't do it unless you have to. If you are seriously concerned to achieve success in partnership, be prepared to nurture and nurture and nurture. (Personal communication from local community representative in a regeneration partnership)

Our conclusion, therefore, is that making partnerships work requires a sophisticated approach. (Huxham and Vangen, 2001)

REFERENCES

Audit Commission, 1998, *A Fruitful Partnership: Effective Partnership Working* (Abingdon: Audit Commission Publications).

Cameron, A. *et al.*, 2000, *Factors Promoting and Obstacles Hindering Joint Working: A Systematic Review* (Bristol South West NHS R&D Directorate).

Huxham, C. and S. Vangen, 2000, 'What Makes Partnerships Work?' in S. Osborne (ed.), *Managing Public Private Partnerships for Public Services* (London: Routledge).

Abstracts

Joint Planning across the Health/Social Services Boundary since 1946, *by Paul Bridgen*
This article reviews the development of post-war policy on the joint planning of health and social services for older people in the context of broader theoretical ideas about inter-organisational collaboration. It identifies the lack of organisational homogeneity and the absence of domain consensus across the health/social services boundary as the main obstacles to progress. However, the article further suggests that, if these problems are to be properly understood, the broader policy context within which joint planning took place must also be investigated. In this regard, the article suggests that central government's attempts to encourage joint planning since the 1960s have repeatedly been hampered by distrust among local agencies of its more general policy intentions in this area.

Conceptual Issues in Inter-Agency Collaboration, *by Wendy Ranade and Bob Hudson*
Inter-agency collaboration – or partnership as it now commonly termed – is central to New Labour's agenda, but the general support for a partnership approach conceals disputes about definitions and approaches. This article begins by examining the shift to more complex and ambitious partnerships in health, social care and regeneration, which require new modes of governance. The three main modes – market, hierarchy and network – are briefly described and contrasted, and located within the recent history of public service development. It is argued that they are best seen as overlain and co-existing, resulting in a hybrid mode of governance which is characterised by tension and contradiction. The article goes on to discuss the issues this raises for real partnerships in trying to understand the collaborative imperative and the barriers to its effective achievement. Although the network mode has its attractions, there are complex issues of membership, management and culture which need to be addressed. It is concluded that hierarchy, markets and networks will co-exist better where each acknowledges its own limits and the strengths of others.

Joint Working: The Health Service Agenda, *by Caroline Glendinning and Anna Coleman*
The purpose of this article is to examine the policy and practice of collaboration between health and local government from a health services

perspective. Within this remit, the authors primarily focus on the area of primary care. Four key elements of the post-1997 policy context are discussed: the move from GP fund-holding to Primary Care Groups and Trusts (PCG/Ts); a shift from treating to preventing illness; a drive for implementation by central government; and an emphasis on collaboration. Within this broad context, there are a number of factors which may support enhanced collaboration: the size, scope, responsibilities and budgets of PCG/Ts may well provide an organisational framework which is supportive of joint working. However, the 'Berlin Wall' between health and social care has proved to be enduring, and there are aspects of the post-1997 policy context which will continue to inhibit effective joint working, in particular centrally designed performance management systems and the dominance by GPs of PCG/Ts.

Health and Local Government Partnerships: The Local Government Policy Context, *by Stephanie Snape*

This article explores partnerships between health and local government from the local government perspective; placing developments between the two sectors within the wider context of the Local Government Modernisation agenda. A number of commentators have argued that developments since 1997 – in particular the emphasis on community leadership and the new power of well-being – have provided local authorities with an exciting opportunity to reclaim a more pivotal role in shaping the health agenda at the local level. Such a role would be based on promoting well-being and a good quality of life, in keeping with the social model of health. In the longer run this reclaimed role could produce a shift in what has become the main boundary between health and local government: the health–social care boundary. The article reviews developments in three key areas: the health–social care boundary; the core components of the Local Government Modernisation Agenda; and the relationship between regeneration and health. The paper concludes that although progress has been made in regeneration and health and there is potential in elements of the Modernisation Agenda that these do not equate to a paradigm shift in local government's perspective on health. Instead, the social care boundary continues to dominate local government's vision of health. Central to this picture of modest progress is the substantial barrier to more radical change provided by the performance management frameworks governing both sectors.

The Health Action Zone Initiative: Lessons from Plymouth, *by Michael Cole*

The article considers the impact of the Health Action Zone (HAZ) in Plymouth through a theory-based evaluation that combines theories of change and realistic evaluation. The study assesses the impact of 37 projects sponsored by this HAZ. The extent to which these projects used a realistic evaluation/theories of change framework and achieved their objectives are evaluated. The impact of these projects on the three main objectives of Plymouth HAZ – developing partnership working; modernising the care system; and tackling health inequalities – is assessed and explanations for the success or failure of specific projects are identified.

Overcoming the Desire for Misunderstanding through Dialogue, *by Paul Hoggett*

The emotional and psychological aspects of joint working are examined in this article, providing a powerful explanation for the continuing difficulties in achieving joined-up government. Drawing on the sociology of community, psycho-dynamics of inter-group behaviour and theories of identity and difference, the author argues that New Labour's vision of an inclusive, consensual, community is inherently flawed; that conflict is a necessary and fundamental aspect of social relations. Indeed, 'splitting' and 'exclusion' are features of geographical, professional and occupational communities. And concepts such as 'relationships-in-the-mind' are valuable in understanding how identities are formed and maintained, and how patterns of conflict, hostility, misunderstanding and non-cooperation develop. Splitting and exclusion are important processes in building group identity, but they can also significantly undermine attempts to develop collaboration between agencies. The answer is for groups to engage in 'conflictual dialogue', addressing openly the misunderstandings created by group identities.

Leading and Managing at the Boundary: Perspectives Created by Joined Up Working, *by Mike Broussine*

Based on a process of action inquiry, this article reflects on the capacities that chief executives need in order to engage effectively with 'joined-up' working. It begins by examining the paradoxical feelings that chief executives can hold about their roles – feeling both powerful and powerless at the same time, for example. By adopting the notion of boundary, it is possible to understand more about the complexities that chief executives need to work with. These boundaries are emotional as much as they are structural. They imply a duality in the role as the chief executive works with the shifting relationships between the organisation and its external world, between organisational and political leadership, and between 'knowing' and 'not knowing'. To be able to work at the boundary, there is a premium on the capacities for sense-making through systemic analysis, for maintaining personal perspective and for seeing leadership as synonymous with learning. In the end, leading at the boundary challenges the chief executive to think from time to time about what he or she stands for as a person.

Notes on Contributors

Paul Bridgen is a lecturer in social policy at the University of Southampton, having previously held research positions at the Universities of Bristol and Oxford. He has published one other article and a book (with Jane Lewis) on 'partnership' working in UK health policy. In the health field, he also has research interests in community empowerment approaches to health promotion, particularly with respect to the New Deal for Communities scheme. Paul is also currently engaged with colleagues in an EU-funded comparative project on private pensions and social inclusion.

Mike Broussine is Director of Research Unit for Organisation Studies at Bristol Business School. He is also Award Leader for the M.Sc. in Leadership and Organisation of Public Services, a programme designed to promote learning across the public, private and voluntary sectors. Main research interests include emotions in organisations, leadership, gender issues, organisational research methods as well as public services management. He undertakes consultancy and action research for organisations, and his experience lies mostly in public services, especially local government.

Michael Cole is Research Associate in the Department of Sociology at the University of Plymouth. He has held academic posts at the Universities of Glamorgan, Northumbria and Exeter. His research interests cover local government, quangos, parliament, devolution, electoral systems and Health Action Zones. He has published in a range of journals including *Local Government Studies*, *The Journal of Legislative Studies*, *Government and Policy*, *Urban Studies*, *Regional and Federal Studies*, *The Political Quarterly* and *Public Policy and Administration*.

Anna Coleman is Research Fellow at the National Primary Care Research and Development Centre, University of Manchester. She has worked on a major longitudinal study of the development of Primary Care Groups and Trusts and a qualitative study of partnerships between NHS and social services. She is currently responsible for a study of the implementation and impact of the new local authority responsibilities for health scrutiny.

Paul Hoggett is Professor of Politics and Director of the Centre for Psycho-Social Studies at the University of the West of England, Bristol. He is interested in bringing together ways of thinking about emotion and identity with concepts of community and the public sphere.

Caroline Glendinning is Professor of Social Policy at the National Primary Care Research and Development Centre, University of Manchester. She leads a programme of research on partnerships between NHS and local authorities. Her wider research interests lie in the fields of social gerontology, disability, community care, informal care and comparative studies of the funding and organisation of services for older people.

Bob Hudson is Principal Research Fellow at the Nuffield Institute for Health, University of Leeds. Prior to that he was Visiting Fellow at the Institute of Health Studies, University of Durtham, and Senior Lecturer in Social Policy, New College, Durham. His main research activity is in the area of integration and partnerships at both professional and organisational levels. His book *The Changing Role of Social Care* was published in 2000. He can be contacted on bob@hudsonb.fsworld.co.uk.

Wendy Ranade was Visiting Research Fellow at the Sustainable Cities Research Institute, University of Northumbria. Prior to that she was Reader in Health Policy at the University. Her most recent research and consultancy activity has been in the field of multi-sectoral partnerships. Now fully retired she is enjoying life as artist, pianist, traveller and child-minder.

Stephanie Snape is a Principal Research Fellow at the Institute of Governance and Public Management (IGPM), University of Warwick. She previously worked as Lecturer at the Institute of Local Government Studies (INLOGOV), University of Birmingham and at the Universities of Salford and Northumbria. Her main research interests include regional policy, new council constitutions, scrutiny, local government reorganisation, the health–local government interface and evaluation theory and practice. She co-edits *Local Government Studies.*

Pat Taylor is a Senior Lecturer in Community Care at the University of the West of England. She was one of the co-sponsors of the ESRC seminar series on which this special edition is based. Her research and teaching interests include public health approaches to primary care, public involvement and partnership working.

Index

Abbott, S., 53, 61
Accountability, 7, 10
Acheson, D., 75
Action inquiry, 128
Alford, D., 118
Alter, C., 38
Anderson, B., 119
Anti-poverty strategies, 75, 99–100
Area Based Initiatives (ABIs), 7, 32, 75, 76, 93–4, 100
Asthana, S., 101

Bate, P., 103, 104
Bauman, Z., 126
Beacon Council scheme, 90
Bed blocking – see hospital discharge
Benington, J., 4
Benjamin, J., 126
Bennis, W., 134
Benson, J.K., 39–40
Best value, 7, 37, 88–9
Better Government for Older People, 65, 81
Bevan, Aneurin, 18
Blair, T., 3, 6
Booth, T.A., 17, 25, 26
Borbon, J., 105
Bosanquet, N., 61
Boundary spanning, 45–7, 132, 135
Bradach, J., 36
Brent, J., 121
Bridgen, P., 11, 20, 21, 22, 23
Brocklehurst, J.C., 21
Broussine, M., 14, 15, 130, 137
Brown, R.G.S., 19
Buffering, 132, 135
Burns, J.M., 134
Burton, J., 38

Calderdale, 25, 26
Callaghan, G.M., 61
Cameron, A., 139
Campbell, F., 74, 75, 76, 78, 81, 92
Campbell, S., 59
Capacity building, 91
Capra, F., 33
Care Trusts, 6, 29, 56, 81
Chandler, D., 123
Charlesworth, J., 40
Children's services – see social services
Clapham, D., 118
Clarke, J., 67, 68, 69

Clarke, K., 61
Clarke, M., 83, 85, 125
Cole, M., 13–14, 99, 100, 103, 105, 106, 107, 108, 109, 110, 111, 112, 113, 114
Colman, A., 57
Collaboration 10–11
    conditions which support effective collaboration, 17
    barriers to collaboration, 40–42
    collaborative advantage, 10–11
    collaborative ladder, 56
    see also partnerships
Commission for Health Improvement (CHI), 7
Community care, 60–61
Community leadership, 76, 83–4
Community safety, 32
Community strategies, 7, 85–6
Comprehensive Performance Assessment (CPA), 89–90
Connell, J.P., 106
Connexions, 7
Coterminosity of boundaries, 24, 63–4
Coulson, A., 112
Cramp, L., 76
Cropper, S., 44
Cross cutting issues – see wicked issues

Dahlgren, G., 77
Davies, J.S., 99
Daum, M., 121, 122, 124
Degeling, P., 45
Departmentalism, 118
Dobson, Frank, 9, 100
Domain consensus, 17, 27
Dowling, B., 54, 58, 67
Dunleavy, A., 57
Duty of partnership – see partnerships

Economic and Social Research Council (ESRC), 1, 2, 139
Eden, C., 42
Education Action Zones (EAZ), 7, 65
Elderly services – see social services

Farey, P., 134
Ferlie, E., 4
Finn, C.B., 42
Flynn, R., 35
Fox, P., 131, 137

Frances, J., 34
French, R., 133, 134
Friedson, E., 118
Friend, J., 45

Gabriel, Y., 129
Garlick, S., 105
Gastor, L., 37
General practitioners, 13, 51, 52, 57, 58, 59, 60, 61, 62, 66–7, 69, 110
General practitioner fund-holding, 12, 51
Giddens, Anthony, 3
Gill, O., 120
Glendinning, C., 8, 11, 12–13, 55, 57, 61, 63, 64, 67, 68
Glennerster, H., 20, 24, 25, 26
Goodman, P.S., 47
Goodwin, N., 52, 58
Governance, 4
Gray, B., 42
Grimshaw, D., 37

Hall, D., 20
Ham, C., 5, 51
Hamer, L., 76, 86, 92
Hardy, B., 40, 41, 44, 47
Harrison, Lyn, 2, 139, 140
Hastings, A., 42, 43
Hatch, M.J., 132
Health Act 1999, 6, 55, 80
    health act flexibilities, 6, 55, 56, 57, 80, 81, 82, 129
Health Action Zones (HAZs), 7, 13, 65, 80, 99–101
    evaluation models, 102–3
    Plymouth Health Action Zone, 13, 99, 101–15
Health and Social Care Act 2001, 6, 56
Health Improvement Plans (HiMPs), 28, 53, 55, 80
Health Improvement and Modernisation Plans (HIMPs), 53, 55, 80
Health inequalities, 13, 52, 53, 69, 75, 99, 101, 105, 110–11
Health promotion, 99
Health scrutiny, 7, 13, 55, 57, 76, 92–3
Healthy city initiative, 75
Healthy Living Centres, 7
Health Visitors, 26
Health–Social Care boundary, 11, 13, 18–20, 73–7, 78–83
Hepatitis C, 109
Higgins, J., 100, 101
Hirschhorn, L., 136
Hiscock, J., 68
Home nursing, 26

Hood, C., 3, 8
Hoggett, P., 14, 15, 36, 126
Holland, W.W., 73
Hospital discharge, 9, 21-23, 26, 54, 56, 68, 91, 112, 113
Hospital Plan 1962, 21–2
Hudson, B., 17, 34, 40, 60, 61, 68, 81, 125, 126
Hunter, D., 73, 75
Huxham, C., 10, 11, 40, 47, 140

Iliffe, S., 54

Jeffers, S., 126
Joint Care Planning Teams (JCPTs), 24, 28, 29, 60
Joint care strategies, 25
Joint commissioning, 62
Joint Consultative Committees (JCCs), 24, 25, 28, 32, 60
Joint finance, 24, 26
    see also pooled budgets
Joint Investment Plans (JIPs), 28, 55, 80
Joint planning, 10, 11, 17–29
Judge, K., 102, 105

Kanter, R.M., 38, 47
Klein, R., 25
'Knowing' and 'not knowing', 14, 133–4
Kouzes, J., 118

Le Grand, J., 47
Leach, S., 93
Leadership, 43, 79
    transactional, 134
    transformational, 134
Leutz, W., 56
Levitas, R., 119
Levitt, T., 134
Lewis, J., 28, 66
Local Agenda 21 initiative, 21, 75
Local Government Act 2000, 6
Local Government Modernisation agenda, 76, 77, 83–93, 95
Local Health and Welfare Plan 1963, 21–2
Local Strategic Partnerships (LSPs), 7, 32, 53, 54, 87
Lorenz, E., 38
Lowndes, V., 36–7, 40, 42, 47

Macintosh, M., 43
Macneil, I., 36
Maoz, I., 124
Marsh, A., 43
Martin, M., 20
Martin, S., 36

Mattesich, P., 44
McCann, J., 47
Medical Officers of Health, 13
Means, R., 23
Metcalfe, L., 38
Milburn, Alan, 13, 100
Models of health, 76, 77–8
  social model of health, 53, 77–8
  medical model of health, 19, 20, 73, 77–8
Moore, M., 4
Myles, S., 61

National Assistance Act 1948, 18
National Health Service Plan for England,
  54, 56, 75, 100
National Priorities Guidance, 80
National Service Frameworks (NSFs), 81
NSF for Older People, 54, 81
Neighbourhood renewal, 32, 94
Networks, 4, 10, 11, 12, 34–8, 42, 45, 46, 47,
  48
New Council Constitutions, 13, 83, 91–3
New Deal for Communities, 32, 65, 76
New Public Management (NPM), 2–3
Newman, I., 93
Newman, J., 4, 8, 15, 44, 54, 56, 99
Nocon, A., 18, 44, 60
North, N., 53, 118, 58, 59, 60, 61, 67

Oral health, 101, 104, 106, 108, 114
Osborne, D., 3
Osborne, S.P., 4–5, 8

Painter, C., 99
Parenting, 108
Partnerships
  barriers to partnership working, 40–42
  co-evolving partnerships, 11, 33, 43
  co-ordinating partnerships, 11, 33
  definitions, 10–11, 129
  duty of partnership, 6, 28, 36, 55, 80
  government levers to encourage
    partnerships, 5–7
  markets, hierarchies and networks, 34–8
  role of local authority chief executive, 14,
    129–38
  transaction costs of partnerships, 47
Paton, C., 52, 53, 55, 100
Pawson, R., 102
Peckham, S., 53, 59, 69
Performance management, 8, 12, 35, 41, 54,
  67–9, 88–91, 93, 95, 96
Pettigrew, A., 44, 47
Plymouth Health Action Zone – see Health
  Action Zones
Pooled budgets, 6, 7, 28, 29, 55, 68, 81, 129

see also health act flexibilities
Power of well-being, 6, 76, 84–5
Pratt, J., 32–3, 36, 37, 38
Primary care, 12, 51–72, 101, 104
Primary Care Groups (PCGs), 12, 52–3, 55,
  57, 80, 109
Primary Care Trusts (PCTs), 6, 12, 52–3, 55,
  57, 80
  size, structure, budget and responsibilities,
    57–60
  partnerships with local authorities, 60–66
  role of general practitioners, 66–7
Private Finance Initiative (PFI), 5
Promoting Independence Partnership Grant,
  80
Public health, 53, 69, 73
  directors of public health, 73
  new public health movement, 75
  public health services, 73
Public Service Agreements (PSAs), 89
Public value, 4

Ranade, W., 1, 11–12, 34, 35, 41–2, 45, 47
Raw, M., 105
Realistic evaluation, 102, 105
Reason, P., 128
Regional Assemblies, 6
Regional Development Agencies (RDAs), 6
Reinventing Government movement, 3
Reticularists, 45–7
Rhodes, R.A.W., 4, 36, 48
Robinson, R., 35
Rogers, S., 19
Royal Commission on Long-Term Care, 29
Rummery, K., 61
Russell, H., 87

Salter, B., 28
Sanderson, I., 113
Schlosberg, D., 125
Scrutiny see Health scrutiny
Seebohm Report, 23–4
Senge, P.M., 133
Sillett, J., 37
Simmel, G., 120
Single Regeneration Budget (SRB), 5
Smith, M., 43
Smoking cessation, 105, 110
Snape, S., 5, 8, 11, 13, 93
Snow, C.C., 38, 46
Social inclusion, 93, 94, 119
Social exclusion, 93, 101
Social services, 6, 9, 11, 19, 20, 21, 23, 25,
  32, 55, 56–7, 58, 60, 62, 63, 64, 65, 67,
  68, 69, 74, 89, 90, 99, 105
  children's services, 101, 104

150 PARTNERSHIPS BETWEEN HEALTH AND LOCAL GOVERNMENT

services for the elderly, 11, 17, 20–23, 26–9,
101, 104, 106–7
see also health–social care divide
Social Services Inspectorate Personal Social
Services Star Ratings, 89–90
Society of Local Authority Chief Executives
(SOLACE), 128, 129, 130, 137
Stakeholder analysis, 42
Stakeholder politics, 3
Stewart, B., 46
Stoker, G., 5
Strategic Health Authorities, 52
Structural interest groups, 118
Substance misuse, 104, 105, 106, 107–8,
109, 110, 112
Sullivan, H., 7, 10, 78–9, 100
Sumner, G., 22
Sure Start, 7, 32, 65

Theories of change (approach to evaluation),
13, 102, 105

Third Way, 1, 3, 32, 51
Tillich, P., 133
Torbert, W.R., 128
Total Purchasing Pilots, 61
Training and Enterprise Councils (TECs), 5

Urban Development Corporations (UDCs), 5

Walby, S., 52
Webb, A., 17, 19
Webb, P., 119
Webster, C., 19, 21, 25, 73
Weiss, C.H., 102
Whitehead, A., 37
Whitfield, D., 37
Whole systems approaches, 100
Wicked issues, 1, 32–3, 43, 48, 125
Wilkin, D., 21, 57, 58, 62, 63, 64, 67, 68
Wistow, G., 9, 17, 25, 26, 27, 29, 35

For Product Safety Concerns and Information please contact our EU
representative GPSR@taylorandfrancis.com
Taylor & Francis Verlag GmbH, Kaufingerstraße 24, 80331 München, Germany

www.ingramcontent.com/pod-product-compliance
Lightning Source LLC
Chambersburg PA
CBHW050528270326
41926CB00015B/3129